Coaching, Mentorship and Leadership in Medicine: Empowering the Development of Patient-Centered Care

Editors

DEAN C. TAYLOR
CAROLYN M. HETTRICH
JONATHAN F. DICKENS
JOE DOTY

CLINICS IN SPORTS MEDICINE

www.sportsmed.theclinics.com

Consulting Editor
MARK D. MILLER

April 2023 • Volume 42 • Number 2

ELSEVIER

1600 John F. Kennedy Boulevard • Suite 1800 • Philadelphia, Pennsylvania, 19103-2899

http://www.theclinics.com

CLINICS IN SPORTS MEDICINE Volume 42, Number 2
April 2023 ISSN 0278-5919, ISBN-13: 978-0-323-93853-2

Editor: Megan Ashdown
Developmental Editor: Diana Grace Ang

Clinics in Sports Medicine (ISSN 0278-5919) is published quarterly by Elsevier Inc., 360 Park Avenue South, New York, NY 10010-1710. Months of issue are January, April, July, and October. Business and Editorial Offices: 1600 John F. Kennedy Blvd., Ste. 1800, Philadelphia, PA 19103-2899. Customer Service Office: 3251 Riverport Lane, Maryland Heights, MO 63043. Periodicals postage paid at New York, NY and additional mailing offices. Subscription prices are $379.00 per year (US individuals), $773.00 per year (US institutions), $100.00 per year (US students), $421.00 per year (Canadian individuals), $953.00 per year (Canadian institutions), $100.00 (Canadian students), $494.00 per year (foreign individuals), $953.00 per year (foreign institutions), and $235.00 per year (foreign students). Foreign air speed delivery is included in all *Clinics* subscription prices. All prices are subject to change without notice. **POSTMASTER:** Send address changes to *Clinics in Sports Medicine*, Elsevier Health Sciences Division, Subscription Customer Service, 3251 Riverport Lane, Maryland Heights, MO 63043. Customer Service (orders, claims, online, change of address): Elsevier Health Sciences Division, Subscription Customer Service, 3251 Riverport Lane, Maryland Heights, MO 63043. **Tel: 1-800-654-2452 (U.S. and Canada); 314-447-8871 (outside U.S. and Canada). Fax: 314-447-8029. E-mail: journalscustomerservice-usa@elsevier.com (for print support); journalsonlinesupport-usa@ elsevier.com (for online support).**

Reprints. For copies of 100 or more of articles in this publication, please contact the Commercial Reprints Department, Elsevier Inc., 360 Park Avenue South, New York, NY 10010-1710. Tel.: 212-633-3874; Fax: 212-633-3820; E-mail: reprints@elsevier.com.

Clinics in Sports Medicine is covered in *MEDLINE/PubMed (Index Medicus) Current Contents/Clinical Medicine, Excerpta Medica,* and *ISI/Biomed.*

Contributors

CONSULTING EDITOR

MARK D. MILLER, MD
S. Ward Casscells Professor, Division of Sports Medicine, Department of Orthopaedic Surgery, University of Virginia, University of Virginia Health System, Team Physician Emeritus, James Madison University, Director, Miller Review Course, Charlottesville, Virginia, USA

EDITORS

DEAN C. TAYLOR, MD
Department of Orthopaedic Surgery, Duke University, Duke University Medical Center, Durham, North Carolina, USA

CAROLYN M. HETTRICH, MD, MPH
N.C.O. New York; Adjunct Professor, University of Iowa, Iowa City, Iowa, USA

JONATHAN F. DICKENS, MD
Duke University, Department of Orthopaedics, Durham, North Carolina, USA; Department of Orthopaedic Surgery, Walter Reed National Military Medical Center, Uniformed Services University of Health Sciences, Bethesda, Maryland, USA; Department of Orthopaedics, Institute of Clinical Sciences, Sahlgrenska Academy, Gothenburg University, Gothenburg, Sweden

JOE DOTY, PhD
Duke University, Executive Director, Feagin Leadership Program, School of Medicine Leadership Program (LEAD), Durham, North Carolina, USA

AUTHORS

PENNY ARCHULETA, MA
Columbia Coaching Certification Program, Fellow, Institute of Coaching, Clinical Instructor, Department of Medicine, University of Colorado, Provider Talent Development Consultant, Children's Hospital Colorado, Littleton, Colorado, USA

RADM BRUCE L. GILLINGHAM, MD
US Navy Bureau of Medicine and Surgery, Falls Church, Virginia, USA; Distinguished Professor, Department of Military and Emergency Medicine, Uniformed Services University of the Health Sciences, Bethesda, Maryland, USA

ERIN S. BARRY, MS
Department of Anesthesiology, Uniformed Services University, Bethesda, Maryland, USA

DAVID N. BERNSTEIN, MD, MBA, MEI
Orthopaedic Surgery Resident Physician, Harvard Combined Orthopaedic Residency Program, Massachusetts General Hospital, Boston, Massachusetts, USA

MEGHAN E. BISHOP, MD
Associate Professor of Orthopaedic Surgery, Rothman Orthopaedic Institute, New York, New York, USA

KEVIN J. BOZIC, MD, MBA
Chair, Professor, Department of Surgery and Perioperative Care, Dell Medical School, The University of Texas at Austin, Austin, Texas, USA

LISA R. COLEMAN, MD, MPH
University of Pennsylvania, Penn Medicine, Philadelphia, Pennsylvania, USA

NEIL E. GRUNBERG, PhD
Department of Military and Emergency Medicine, Uniformed Services University, Bethesda, Maryland, USA

F. WINSTON GWATHMEY, MD
Associate Professor, Department of Orthopaedic Surgery, University of Virginia, University of Virginia Health System, Charlottesville, Virginia, USA

LEAH D. HOUDE, PhD
Chief Learning Officer, PwC-US

SHARON K. HULL, MD, MPH
Professional Certified Coach (ICF), Adjunct Professor, Department of Family Medicine, The University of North Carolina at Chapel Hill, School of Medicine, Founder and CEO, Metta Solutions, LLC, Durham, North Carolina, USA

FRANCIS H. KEARNEY, LTG (ret), USA
Thayer Leadership, West Point, New York, USA

CAPT CHRISTOPHER A. KURTZ, MD
US Navy Bureau of Medicine and Surgery, Falls Church, Virginia, USA; Assistant Professor, Department of Surgery, Uniformed Services University of the Health Sciences, Bethesda, Maryland, USA

JOE LEBOEUF, COL, US Army, Retired, PhD
Professor of the Practice of Management Emeritus, Duke University, Fuqua School of Business, LeadershipMatters LLC, Charlotte, North Carolina, USA

MARIANNE LEPRE-NOLAN, PCC
President, Marianne Lepre-Nolan, Inc

LANCE E. LECLERE, MD
Associate Professor of Orthopaedic Surgery, Vanderbilt University Medical Center, Nashville, Tennessee, USA

JOHN E. MCMANIGLE, MD
Department of Military and Emergency Medicine, Uniformed Services University, Bethesda, Maryland, USA

MARK D. MILLER, MD
S. Ward Casscells Professor, Division of Sports Medicine, Department of Orthopaedic Surgery, University of Virginia, University of Virginia Health System, Team Physician Emeritus, James Madison University, Director, Miller Review Course, Charlottesville, Virginia, USA

DARYL J. NELSON, MS, LAT, ATC
New England Patriots, Foxboro, Massachusetts, USA

FRANCIS G. O'CONNOR, MD, MPH, COL (ret), MC, USA
Professor, Department of Military and Emergency Medicine, Uniformed Services University of the Health Sciences, Bethesda, Maryland, USA

CAPT MATTHEW T. PROVENCHER, MD, MBA, MC, USNR (Ret.)
Steadman Philippon Research Institute, The Steadman Clinic, Vail, Colorado, USA

JOANN FARRELL QUINN, PhD, MBA
Director of SELECT Competency Assessment, Department of Medical Education, TGH-USF People Development Institute, Academic Director, Muma College of Business, Associate Professor, University of South Florida Tampa, Florida, USA

ERIC B. SCHOOMAKER, MD, PhD
Department of Military and Emergency Medicine, Uniformed Services University, Bethesda, Maryland, USA

POONAM SHARMA, MD
Professional Certified Coach (ICF), Chair, Department of Pathology, Creighton University School of Medicine, CHI Health, Founder of Sharma Coaching and Consulting LLC, Omaha, Nebraska, USA

SANYIN SIANG, MBA
Executive Director, Fuqua/Coach K Center on Leadership and Ethics, Pratt School of Engineering, Professor, Duke University, Durham, North Carolina, USA

ALYSSA M. STEPHANY, MD, MS
Professional Certified Coach (ICF), Director, Physician-Provider Organizational Support and Director, Leadership Center for Physicians, Children's Mercy Kansas City, Associate Professor, University of Missouri-Kansas City, School of Medicine, Associate Professor, University of Kansas School of Medicine, Kansas City, Missouri, USA

PATRICK J. SWEENEY, COL, Retired, US Army, PhD
Professor of the Practice of Management, Executive Director, Allegacy Center for Leadership and Character, School of Business, Wake Forest University, Winston-Salem, North Carolina, USA

ERICA D. TAYLOR, MD, MBA, FAAOS, FAOA
Duke University School of Medicine, Duke Health, Wake Forest, North Carolina, USA

ROBIN WEST, MD
President, Inova MSK Service Line, Lead Team Physician, Washington Nationals, Associate Professor, Georgetown University Medical Center, Associate Professor, Uniformed Services University of Health Sciences, Professor of Medical Education, UVA School of Medicine, Inova Campus, Fairfax, Virginia, USA

JAMES M. WHALEN, MSEd, ATC
New England Patriots, Foxboro, Massachusetts, USA

RYAN J. WHALEN, BS, CSCS
Steadman Philippon Research Institute, Vail, Colorado, USA

BOBBIE ANN ADAIR WHITE, EdD, MA
Associate Professor, Department of Health Professions Education, School of Healthcare Leadership, MGH (Massachusetts General Hospital) Institute of Health Professions, Charlestown Navy Yard, Boston, Massachusetts, USA

Contents

Executive coaches use a disciplined process to enable people to uncover why they are getting their current results and stimulate them to identify new ideas to achieve different results in the future. Unlike mentors, coaches do not give direction or advice. A coach might offer examples of what others have done in similar situations but only in service to idea generation, not recommendations. Data is key. Coaches typically gather information through assessments or interviews to give clients new insights. Clients learn about their deficiencies and strengths, their brand, how they work with teams, and glean unvarnished advice. Mindset matters. Anyone coerced into coaching might be frustrated about their situation and, therefore, be less open to honestly discovering the source of their discomfort and uncovering new possibilities through coaching. Courage is crucial. Being open to coaching can be daunting, yet with a willing mindset, the insights and results can be compelling.

Professional coaching can support individuals and organizations in four ways: (1) improving provider experience of working in health care, (2) supporting provider role and career development, (3) helping build team effectiveness, and (4) building an organizational coaching culture. There is evidence about effectiveness of coaching in business, and an increasing body of literature, including small randomized, controlled trials, supporting use of coaching in health care. This article summarizes the framework for professional coaching, describes ways professional coaching can support the four processes above, and provides case scenarios that contextualize understanding of how professional coaching can be of benefit.

From the increase in telehealth to the expansion of private investors to the growth of transparency (both price and patient outcomes) and value-based care initiatives, health-care delivery is rapidly changing. At the same time, demand for musculoskeletal care continues to rapidly increase, with more than 1.7 billion people globally suffering from musculoskeletal conditions, yet burnout is a major concern and growing since the onset COVID-19 global pandemic. When taken together, these factors have a major impact on the health-care delivery environment and pose enormous challenges and increased stressors on orthopedic surgeons and their teams. Coaching can help.

alterations, and new situations. Many perspectives, models, theories, and steps have been offered to optimize change. Some approaches emphasize organizational change, whereas others focus on responses of individuals to change. With regard to leading change in health care, it is important to enhance well-being among health-care professionals and patients and to improve organizational and system best practices. To achieve optimal health-care changes, this article draws from several business-focused approaches to change leadership, psychological models, and the authors' Leader-Follower Framework (LF2).

Emotional intelligence (EI) has gained popularity and is being seen as a necessity, spreading beyond the business world, and becoming universal. In that shift, medicine and medical education have started to see the importance. This is evident in mandatory curriculum and accreditation requirements. EI includes 4 primary domains with several subcompetencies under each domain. This article outlines several of the subcompetencies necessary for success as a physician, competencies that can be honed with targeted professional growth. Empathy, communication, conflict management, burnout, and leadership are discussed in an application way to help identify importance of and how to improve each.

Diversity, equity, and inclusion (DEI) increases performance through input of differing ideas and perspectives, leading to outcomes such as increased diagnostic accuracy, patient satisfaction, quality of care, and retention of talent. DEI can be difficult to establish due to the presence of unaddressed biases and ineffective policies against discrimination and noninclusive behaviors. Nevertheless, these complexities can be overcome through the integration of principles of DEI into the standard operations of health care, incentivizing DEI efforts through leadership curriculums, and highlighting the value proposition of diversifying our workforce as a critical asset to success.

The still-evolving global pandemic has accelerated changes in how we work, how we lead, and how we interact. The power dynamic that once drove institutions has shifted to an infrastructure and operating framework encouraging new employee expectations, including the humanization of leadership from those in power. Trends in the corporate world show organizations have shifted to operational frameworks with humanized leadership models: leader-as-coach and leader-as-mentor.

Coaching, mentorship, and leadership are all paramount for the creation of a championship-winning football team. Looking back and studying the great coaches of professional football provides valuable insight into the qualities and the characteristics they possessed and how that impacted their leadership. Many of the great coaches from this game have instilled team standards and a culture that led to unprecedented success and sprouted into many other great coaches and leaders. Leadership at all levels of an organization is essential to consistently achieve a championship-caliber team.

The military provides a valuable resource for the civilian medical education sector to potentially model or adopt strategies used to train emerging leaders. The Department of Defense has a long tradition of cultivating leaders, espousing a culture that emphasizes a value system that promotes selfless service and integrity. In addition to leadership training, and a fostered value system, the military additionally trains leaders to use a defined military decision-making process. This article identifies and shares lessons learned in how the military structures and focuses to accomplish the mission, and develops and invests in military leadership training.

Patient-centered care is safe and eliminates preventable patient harm. Sports medicine teams that understand and apply the principles of high reliability, as demonstrated by high-performing communities in the US Navy, will provide safer, higher-quality care. Sustaining high-reliability performance is challenging. Leadership is essential to creating an accountable but psychologically safe environment fostering active engagement by all team members and resisting complacency. Leaders who invest the time and energy to create the appropriate culture and who model the required behaviors enjoy an exponential return on their investment in terms of professional satisfaction and the delivery of truly patient-centered, safe, high-quality care.

Similar to elite athletes, surgeons use their skills on a daily basis but coaching for skillset refinement is not common among surgeons. Surgeon coaching has been proposed a method by which surgeons can gain insight into their performance and optimize their practice. However, many barriers exist to surgeon coaching such as logistics, time, cost, and pride. Ultimately, the tangible improvement in surgeon performance, the elevation of surgeon well-being, the optimization of the practice, and better patient outcomes support a wider implementation of surgeon coaching for surgeons at all stages of their career.

CLINICS IN SPORTS MEDICINE

THE CLINICS ARE AVAILABLE ONLINE!
Access your subscription at:
www.theclinics.com

CLINICS IN SPORTS MEDICINE

FORTHCOMING ISSUES

July 2023
On-the-Field Emergencies
Eric McCarty, Sourav K. Poddar, and Alex Ebinger, Editors

October 2023
Acromioclavicular Injuries and Sternoclavicular Injuries in Athletes
Katherine J. Coyner, Editor

January 2024
Equality, Diversity, and Inclusion in Sports Medicine
Joel Boyd and David T. Helland, Editor

RECENT ISSUES

January 2023
Advances in the Treatment of Rotator Cuff Tears
Brian C. Werner, Editor

October 2022
Pediatric & Adolescent Knee Injuries: Evaluation, Treatment & Rehabilitation
Matthew D. Milewski, Editor

July 2022
Sports Cardiology
Peter N. Dean, Editor

SERIES OF RELATED INTEREST

Orthopedic Clinics
Physical Medicine and Rehabilitation Clinics
Foot and Ankle Clinics
Hand Clinics
Physician Assistant Clinics

THE CLINICS ARE AVAILABLE ONLINE
Access your subscription at
www.theclinics.com

Foreword

Put Me in Coach!

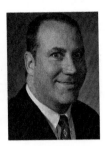

Mark D. Miller, MD
Consulting Editor

Ten years ago, when I was the Program Director for the American Orthopaedic Society for Sports Medicine (AOSSM), I came across a 2011 article by Atul Gawande in *The New Yorker*. Dr Gawande invited a senior surgeon into his operating room to observe his practice and provide the requested feedback. The idea intrigued me, and we put together a symposium for the 2013 AOSSM Annual Meeting on coaching. The details are included in the final article in this issue, but suffice it to say, the symposium was a success. Ten years later, as President of the AOSSM, I discussed resurrecting this symposium for the 2023 meeting with my program directors, and we decided to expand the focus to include mentorship and leadership. To this end, I have been closely following the development of the Feagin Leadership Program by my colleague and friend, Dr Dean Taylor. This program, which began in 2008, was developed to improve leadership training within medical education. So...who better to guest edit an issue on this topic for *Clinics in Sports Medicine*?

It took some convincing, and perhaps Dean agreed to do this largely as a favor to me. So...thank you! Dr Taylor wisely invited some coeditors with coaching and leadership experience. Thank you, Dr Hettrich, former chair of the Emerging Leaders program at AOSSM; Dr Dickens, former West Point surgeon and fellowship program director; and Joe Doty, PhD, Executive Director of the Feagin Leadership Program and former deputy director for the Center of Army Professional Ethic. They invited a very talented group of authors to share their secrets on coaching, mentoring, and leadership. The result is a fantastic treatise on this topic that I encourage all to read cover to cover.

As we bring many of these lessons to the AOSSM Annual Meeting this summer (July 13–16, 2023 in Washington, DC), I hope that this issue of *Clinics in Sports Medicine* will serve as a playbook for the symposium on this topic. I am excited to see how Dr Taylor,

Clin Sports Med 42 (2023) xiii–xiv
https://doi.org/10.1016/j.csm.2023.01.002
0278-5919/23/© 2023 Published by Elsevier Inc.

who is the next AOSSM President, takes this to the next level the following year in Denver, Colorado.

Mark D. Miller, MD
Division of Sports Medicine
Department of Orthopaedic Surgery
University of Virginia
James Madison University
400 Ray C. Hunt Drive, Suite 330
Charlottesville, VA 22908-0159, USA

E-mail address:
MDM3P@hscmail.mcc.virginia.edu

Preface

Coaching, Mentorship, and Leadership in Medicine: Empowering the Development of Patient-Centered Care

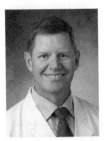

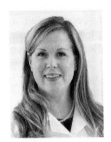

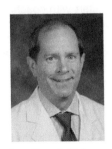

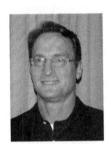

Dean C. Taylor, MD   Carolyn M. Hettrich, MD, MPH   Jonathan F. Dickens, MD   Joe Doty, PhD

Editors

Health care today is complex and challenging. The daily challenges of exponentially expanding medical knowledge, upheavals from the COVID-19 pandemic, and ever-changing economic pressures, to name a few, weigh constantly on all of us engaged in caring for patients. Our expertise and knowledge grow exponentially; innovations multiply; and technological applications expand. With all these advances, why is the public's satisfaction with their health care and health care delivery *decreasing* over time? The answer—the development of our interpersonal and team-building skills and advances in how we care for our fellow humans—both patients and colleagues—have not kept pace with our technical development.

How do we make health care better? We make health care better by preparing ourselves for the leadership challenges that we face now and in the future. We learn to develop better interpersonal and team-building skills, to cultivate exceptional patient-centered teams, and to live lives that are rewarding and resilient.

How can we excel at our jobs while also decreasing burnout and increasing personal happiness? We can learn that through mentorship and coaching to be more effective leaders, and having these resources can decrease stress that is associated with decision making and implementing change. Coaching can also help to thoughtfully define priorities to help leaders to protect their time away from work and increase personal happiness.

Clin Sports Med 42 (2023) xv–xviii
https://doi.org/10.1016/j.csm.2023.01.001
0278-5919/23/© 2023 Published by Elsevier Inc.

sportsmed.theclinics.com

How do we accomplish these goals? The simple answer is through developing ourselves as leaders through coaching, mentorship, and intentional leadership development so that we can collectively address the complex challenges of health care. Everyone has a responsibility to lead in health care. In medicine, we can better meet this responsibility and make health care better by continuously developing our leadership skills and intentionally teaching leadership skills to the next generation of medical leaders. Furthermore, by being fully engaged in this teaching process, established leaders will not only grow their leadership skills but also reap the invaluable rewards and satisfaction that come with serving their honorable profession and those who will follow in their footsteps while decreasing burnout.

In this special issue of *Clinics in Sports Medicine* dedicated to leadership and leadership development, we start with coaching, and how coaching accelerates professional and personal leadership development. Lepre-Nolan and Houde focus on coaching as a powerful process for developing leadership skills. Hull and colleagues provide specific insight on how coaching can effectively improve medicine and health care through enhanced leadership. Bernstein and Bozic focus on how executive coaching enhances the specialty of orthopedic surgery and can help to avoid burnout.

As the authors of this special issue clearly articulate, coaching and mentorship are complementary in leadership development, and although sometimes incorrectly used synonymously, they are significantly different concepts. In our section on mentorship, we explore these differences and how mentors and mentees can make the most of their mentorship opportunities. LeBeouf and Sweeney share their mentorship insights from the business world. From a medical perspective, West contributes insights on how to be a good mentor and what to look for in mentees, and LeClere and Bishop contribute insights on how to get the most out of mentorship from mentees' perspectives.

As we examine how coaching and mentorship accelerate leadership development, it is important to define the term "leadership," and specifically, "leadership in health care." Our definition of *leadership in health care is the ability to influence others for the benefit of patients and patient populations.* Through more effective, ethical leadership, *all* health care will benefit.

The question is, "How do we arrive at more effective, ethical leadership?" The answer is, by emphasizing and teaching recognized skills that will lead to improved health care leadership competencies. Hargett and colleagues[1] helped define what those leadership competencies are and developed a model that can be used as a framework for teaching leadership skills (**Fig. 1**). Patient-centeredness is intentionally positioned centrally not as a core competency but rather as a core *principle.* The core competencies are emotional intelligence, positioned at the top of the model as the "keystone" to effective health care leadership; service and integrity, positioned at the base as foundational competencies; and critical thinking and teamwork, positioned as pillars or struts to provide structure to leadership education.

This special issue explores in-depth these leadership competencies. Quinn and White critically examine why emotional intelligence is essential for leadership in health care in order to care for patients as well as colleagues. Coleman and Taylor help us develop all five leadership competencies in their reflections on the importance of diversity, equity, and inclusion for effective, ethical leadership. Critical thinking, emotional intelligence, service, integrity, and teamwork are also all highlighted in the insights of Gruenberg and colleagues in their investigation on leading change as seen through the lens of their Leader-Follower Framework.

In many ways, health care is behind other fields in leadership. For example, health care remains a very hierarchical profession when increasing complexity calls for more

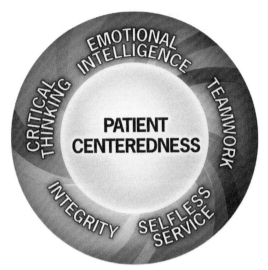

Fig. 1. Duke Healthcare Leadership Model. (Copyright 2017 Dean C. Taylor, MD, all rights reserved.)

distributed leadership that empowers all in health care to address challenges at all levels appropriate to their experience and position. To help us advance our leadership skills in health care, we have assembled experts from the business world, athletics, and the military to share their lessons learned. Siang provides a wealth of insight from the business world. Whalen and colleagues share insights from professional football applicable to coaching, mentorship, and leadership in health care. Military leadership has many parallels with health care leadership. O'Connor and Kearney share lessons learned from an Army perspective that can enhance our leadership in health care. Gillingham and Kurtz provide us with a view from the Navy on developing highly reliable organizations so that we can more successfully create and advance health care organizations.

In concluding this special issue of *Clinics in Sports Medicine*, we have dedicated an article on coaching specifically in *sports medicine* by Gwathmey and Miller. Gwathmey and Miller tie together the concepts of coaching, mentorship, and leadership with examples from the sports medicine field.

We hope that you enjoy this special issue. Our goal is to improve health care through more effective and intentional leadership. The lessons learned and shared in this special issue will empower all of us to continue to develop our health care leadership competencies and prepare us for the current and future leadership challenges involved in delivering effective, ethical patient-centered care.

Dean C. Taylor, MD
Department of Orthopaedic Surgery
Duke University
Duke University Medical Center
Box 3615
Durham, NC 27710, USA

Carolyn M. Hettrich, MD, MPH

Jonathan F. Dickens, MD
Department of Orthopaedics
Duke University
Durham, NC 27710, USA

Joe Doty, PhD
Duke University
DUMC Box 3615
Durham, NC 27710, USA

E-mail addresses:
dean.taylor@duke.edu (D.C. Taylor)
carolyn.hettrich@gmail.com (C.M. Hettrich)
jonathan.dickens@duke.edu (J.F. Dickens)
joseph.doty@duke.edu (J. Doty)

REFERENCE

1. Hargett CW, Doty JP, Hauck JN, et al. Developing a model for effective leadership in healthcare: a concept mapping approach. J Healthc Leadersh 2017;9:69–78.

Coaching

Lessons from Executive Coaches: Why You Need One

Marianne Lepre-Nolan, P.C.C.[a],*, Leah D. Houde, PhD[b,1]

KEYWORDS

- Coaching • Executive Coaching • Leadership • Growth • Transformation

KEY POINTS

- Executive coaching is about helping people identify both why they are getting the results they are currently experiencing and about helping them identify new paths to achieving different results in the future.
- Coaching has made its way beyond the boardroom and into the clinic.
- Mindset is an essential component in a coaching relationship with some mindsets more conducive to success than others.
- Assessments can provide insights, a common vocabulary, and references toward more compelling coaching conversations.
- Stories illustrate how coaching comes to life in practice.

Coaching as a concept has been around for thousands of years, and at its most basic definition refers to a relationship where one individual is in some way training or instructing another toward an outcome, usually improved skill or performance. However, the notion of executive coaching is a relatively recent phenomenon, first appearing in the management literature in the 1950s as a way to develop employees through apprenticeship-type relationships,[1] expanding in the 1960s as part of the Human Potential Movement,[2] and gaining broader popularity in the 1980s.[3] In fact, the field continues to grow with total global revenue from coaching in 2019 estimated at more than US $2.8 billion, a 21% increase over 2015.[4] So, what is all the buzz about?

The International Coaching Federation defines executive coaching as "partnering with clients in a thought-provoking and creative process that inspires them to maximize their personal and professional potential. The process of coaching often unlocks previously untapped sources of imagination, productivity, and leadership." Executive coaching has already made its way beyond the boardroom into the clinic; one study found that physicians who receive executive coaching covering topics such as professional fulfillment, leadership development, improving efficiency, self-care, cultivating

[a] Marianne Lepre-Nolan, Inc.; [b] PwC-US
[1] Present address: 1060 West Forest Hills Blvd, Durham, NC 27707, USA.
* Corresponding author. 57 Seaside South Court, Key West, FL 33040
E-mail address: Marianne@mleprenolan.com

Clin Sports Med 42 (2023) 185–193
https://doi.org/10.1016/j.csm.2022.11.005
0278-5919/23/© 2022 Elsevier Inc. All rights reserved.

community, and integrating personal and professional life has helped to alleviate burnout.[5]

Many organizations emphasize the importance of coaching for employees' career progression and often put formal programs in place to match individuals with "coaches." In this instance, however, we suggest that these organizations are creating mentorship relationships—where an experienced guide gives advice to less-experienced individuals based on what worked well in their own careers. At its most effective, the mentor considers a mentee's context and aspirations but at its heart, mentoring is an advisory relationship.

Executive coaching, differentiated from mentoring, is about helping individuals identify goals they would like to achieve and then discover the most effective path to take to achieve those goals. A coaching colleague of ours uses a metaphor to describe it: imagine you are in a boat traveling down a river you have never traveled on before, and it is dark. A mentor would tell you which way to steer based on having traveled this river extensively. A coach would hold a lantern up in the bow of the boat to illuminate the river so that you could see what lies ahead and which path you would like to take. Coaches use a disciplined approach that enables their coachees to uncover both why they are getting their current results, as well as stimulates how the coachee can use new ideas to achieve different results in the future. Notwithstanding that coaches often help their coachees see new possibilities, the process is about reflection and self-discovery rather than advising or even skill building (which falls into the realm of performance coaching).

MINDSETS THAT AFFECT COACHING

Individuals seek out executive coaching for many reasons, and although anyone can benefit from coaching, there are some mindsets that are more conducive to progress than others. We like to think about motivation for being coached along 2 axes: urgency and willingness. Let us explore all the combinations (**Fig. 1**).

Low Urgency/Low Willingness—Apathetic

Unfortunately, this is often someone who has been "assigned" coaching as a final attempt to keep them at an organization when their performance has degraded. These people often show up in coaching conversations as surly, or even angry and can even be apathetic about keeping their jobs. Often, they feel "wronged" by their organization, possibly having been passed over for promotions. They may have erroneous thoughts about why others get ahead while they do not move forward in their careers. Sometimes, these are individuals who are close to retirement and have lost the spark to deliver high performance, and sometimes people in this category are not necessarily close to retirement, but are on performance improvement plans where the organization thinks it needs to make one final attempt at turning things around before firing

Willingness

	Begrudging	Total engagement
Urgency	Apathetic	Transformational growth

Fig. 1. Urgency and willingness.

them. Whatever the case, they need an experienced executive coach to help them find possibility past the walls they have erected around themselves. It is not unusual for these individuals to make little progress through a coaching experience without having the willingness to get out of denial.

High Urgency/Low Willingness—Begrudging

These are individuals who wake up one morning and realize that their career has stalled or is even disintegrating, and often they really do not know why. Maybe they have been doing the same things they have always done, but the competencies that made them brilliant five years ago may actually work against them now. Perhaps they are overusing a strength constantly and in situations where it is inappropriate, and it has become a liability. Often below the surface, they sense something is "off," or they may actively recognize something is very wrong! Alternatively, they may have been approached to be down-leveled or conversely have been given more responsibility but applied the old tools unsuccessfully. Their challenge is they cannot figure out what to do, or they keep doing the wrong things. Anxiety may underpin their days— and many nights. They come to coaching begrudgingly because it might be the only answer to keep their job or to get themselves out of the malaise.

High Urgency/High Willingness—Total Engagement

We find lots of energy here! These individuals typically seek out coaching for themselves although some have coaching suggested for them, but even these "nudged" folks are excited about what they can gain from the coaching experience. Perhaps they have a new project, or maybe they are launching a new endeavor. Many are entrepreneurial and are highly motivated, often looking for someone with whom to test their thinking and their approaches to new challenges or contexts. Our biggest challenge as coaches with these individuals is keeping things focused because conversations are almost raucous with possibilities. The vast majority of these interactions reap fruitful outcomes because the individual's energy, time, and efforts are fully engaged.

Low Urgency/High Willingness—Transformational Growth

These are some of our favorite coaching interactions. These coachees are often people who have experienced coaching or have a long-time relationship with a coach. There is a free form and sweeping nature to the conversations. Transformation is in the air—there is a sense of movement but there may be no particular goal or project. Sometimes, people in this box are looking ahead to a different time of life, maybe maternity leave will happen at some point, or a second career is being planned in parallel with the current one. Retirement from the work that has been done most of a person's life may be on the horizon, and they want to brainstorm about what is next. Maybe someone wants to "play" with a new skill or test a competency that heretofore has not been needed in their current work. These kinds of conversations can also take place on retreats or off-site meetings where introspection is part of the experience. Whatever the case, even while there is not a pressing goal or vision of the future being activated, often these relationships result in quantum leaps for coachees as they openly explore possibilities for new and exciting futures.

THE VALUE OF DATA IN COACHING

Regardless of a person's motivation to be coached, the process is a reflective one where coachees are supported by their coaches through a process of self-discovery. In his bestseller *The Soul's Code*, James Hillman proposed that our calling in life is in-born and that it is our mission to realize its imperatives over the course of our lives. His "acorn theory" suggests that implanted within everyone is a unique and innate image that "gives us our sense of calling in life, forms our most essential character, and gives us the particularity we feel about ourselves."[6]

So, when is the right time to hold up the mirror and try to use the reflected light to identify that particularity and learn more scientifically your strengths, weaknesses, and motivations? Typically, when you are motivated to do so! For someone who is approaching coaching with keen interest or even outright zeal, marked by a desire for growth and transformation (see **Fig. 1**), the right psychometric assessment can provide information that is revelatory. At the most basic level, an assessment can provide both client and coach with a common vocabulary and references for inflection points in compelling conversations. As well, assessments often offer insights into a client's patterns of behavior both personally and within organizations. For example, if a client has low scores in patience, tact, self-awareness, and self-restraint with high scores in verbal acuity, assertiveness, self-expression, and decisiveness, they might be unintentionally brusque and may be leaving trails of unmotivated, hurt, and confused colleagues in their wake without even realizing their effect.

We all have Achilles' heels, and it is optimum to use an assessment to understand our proclivities and why we might be resistant to change during or as a prelude to the coaching process. An Achilles' heel is an apt metaphor—the term describes a weakness in spite of overall strength, which can lead to a downfall. For a coaching candidate, assessments may indeed bring to light exactly where they have both strengths and blind spots.

LESSONS FROM THE FIELD

With an understanding of what executive coaching is and some of the components that can make it a successful endeavor, you may be asking yourself, "how might this help me?" It may be illuminating to read about coaching that your authors have engaged in to see how it actually plays out in real life. In our final section, we share some stories from our own coaching practices to help illustrate how these ideas can come to life in practice. Perhaps you will see yourself in one of the vignettes.

Lesson One: Denial is a Derailer

Jim wanted one thing: a promotion to what in professional services firms is known as Managing Director (MD). He hired me as his coach to learn what criteria his firm held for becoming one because he thought he had gone as far as he could on his own gleaning specific information about what the role entailed and what was holding him back. Thus, he wanted a coach to get a more informed view. MD is a significant step and can be the last stop that crowns a stellar career. It is often akin to partner, as, an MD holds both people and client leadership responsibilities and the associated compensation, but without the ownership realities of partnership. Firms are apprenticeships that value those entering at the bottom rung who have the highest perceived future value. People who become part of a professional services firm or any other partnership are sponsored and mentored their entire careers toward being an integral part of the engine of financial and professional growth at their firms. Those who put "the interests of the firm ahead of their own needs" are more aligned with the partners of the firm andthus the partnership has "higher odds that it will achieve its objectives over time."[7,8]

Similar to most people who engage in coaching sponsored by their organization, Jim engaged in a 360-feedback process, and received personality data gleaned from an assessment matched to his needs. Jim chose over a dozen of his constituents for me to interview for the 360-feedback process and learned more about himself through the personality assessment. The results highlighted that he was technically brilliant but was challenged by low self-awareness, low other-awareness, and an intensely competitive personality. He also struggled to accept these insights as I held up the mirror of the prevailing data. Patterns emerged that made it apparent he was being held back by an oblivious insensitivity to others.

During the feedback-gathering process, Jim was cited by a managing partner as being a poor collaborator and a terrible people manager—two well-regarded scientists had left the firm while working on his teams. Jim had a voracious competitiveness that led to an ignorant approach to leadership with an inability to see shades of grey when situations were not binary. Through my interviews with his constituents the picture was clear—he was a brilliant individual contributor who could solve problems that discouraged others and was a strong advocate for groups and teams, but people worked in fear of his condescending and intimidating style. The feedback was emphatic and specific, but Jim was unable to see himself as others saw him. Even when the mirror was held up with verbatim quotes that described his affect, he denied his behavior had anything to do with not being promoted. "Yes, but..." was a frequent interjection in our conversations. He was issued an interview report of more than 20 pages but could not cross the bridge between how others saw him and how he saw himself. The promotion was not rendered, and Jim remained frustrated and declined further coaching feeling the problem lay elsewhere. His technical success and promotability was undermined by his abrasiveness and lack of self-awareness but more impactfully, Jim was held back from evolving by a mindset of resistance and defensiveness. Until he could accept the need for both change and for help making those changes, he was a prisoner of his own making.

Lesson Two: Baptism by Fire—Epiphany

When the legal office of a company reaches out to a coach, it is often because there is an imminent "save" situation. In baseball, a save is awarded to the relief pitcher who finishes a game for the winning team. Tom is typical of someone an organization determines is worth the save. These people are often known for their rainmaking or technical skill. Tom fit the bill; he was a brilliant technician and a client favorite but had a formal complaint registered against him from a chronic complainer. This frequent flyer of complaints had Tom in their cross hairs. There was a measure of truth in the accusations, but they were greatly inflated. He knew his part in the situation was not egregious but the firm needed to go through the investigation process all the same. When I met Tom, he was defensive and confused, with our conversations circling around the theme "nobody understands me." No one doubted he was very smart but as well as his complaint woes, his colleagues were tired of him telling them about his acumen and expertise. His orientation toward coaching was definitely in the begrudging box. He was in a change or die situation—if the investigation swung the wrong way, his job could be on the line. His fear about the charges was palpable and he had already lost real money over the situation which drove his, although reluctant, willingness to be coached. His fear got him past his defensiveness.

As his coach, I performed interviews and a personality assessment. The report from the interviews was scathing—Tom was leaving trails of bruised people in his wake. He was tone deaf to anyone trying to give him feedback in the usual channels, and he did not understand that his impact did not match his intentions.

We started the process by absorbing the results of the personality assessment. Among the many insights that came from the data, it showed that he had little patience or tact, and importantly that he had little self-respect. One quote from the interviews that resonated with him and helped him see the impact he was having on others was that he was an "egomaniac with an inferiority complex." The technician in him loved that the assessment gave him raw data about himself over a broad spectrum of traits. As an expert in certain aspects of computer science, he needed data—real, raw, data—about himself. Thus, the objective assessment information combined with the subjective interview opinions were the perfect combination for a reflective person to try to understand his situation. The data helped him uncover why he was being misperceived, which catalyzed his willingness to change. He courageously spoke with and thanked his constituents who participated in the interviews. Then we went to work. With the right mix of data, discussion, reflection, and coaching, he was able to understand the root causes of his issues and set the intentions and mitigation plan to become the leader he always had the potential to be.

Lesson Three: Delighting in the Realizations of Progress

I had been subcontracting with a professional services organization for many years when one of its own leaders, Elizabeth, reached out to me for coaching. She had been active in a variety of leadership roles—an office leadership role where she was responsible for market development as well as staff morale, and a global functional leadership role that landed her on the executive leadership team. Moreover, although she was successful in both roles, she had realized that the internal focus of each was deenergizing for her and she wanted to go back to serving external clients. However, she still viewed herself as a leader and wanted to continue leading within the organization. Therefore, the question became, "Where and how are you a leader without a formal title as such?"

We agreed to have her complete the assessment that best mapped to her challenges, and the results debunked her notion of what it meant to be a thought leader (which to her had always been writing and publishing). The assessment showed she had inordinate skill as a thought leader in conversations. Reflecting on this data and processing it through our coaching discussions opened up a new possibility for Elizabeth that she had not seen for herself—that her skill and expertise was better expressed through dialog, not the written word. For Elizabeth, the data made this idea legitimate.

With new insight into her own preferences and how those epiphanies were more effectively expressed in her work to enable high impact, Elizabeth also reflected on what parts of the work were energizing for her. Using those energizers catalyzed her to shape a new service for her organization to provide to clients. She recognized that she could lead through the work without a formal job title and became one of the highest producing professionals in her organization, coaching and growing others to do the work alongside her, and building strong relationships in the market. These combined allowed her to progress her career past a traditional path in her current organization.

Because Elizabeth continued flexing these new muscles and deepening this freshly realized skill set by applying them in new contexts, the culture and work of her current organization was shifting. She wanted to pursue deep advisory relationships with her clients but the organization was moving toward lower cost and higher volume work. Our work together gave her the confidence to chase and retain the advisory work and believe that she could go beyond being a "big fish in a small pond." She left that organization and was able to represent herself as a thought leader capable of strategically advising clients and, as a result, landed a C-level role at a large professional services firm. The coaching process helped Elizabeth reframe her strengths, which unlocked new possibilities, and ultimately served as jet fuel to propel her career forward.

Lesson 4: Transformation

Changes for Tom, aforementioned in our Lesson Two, came fast and furious because he applied himself wholeheartedly to our coaching strategy. He had become a leader who was finally realizing his full potential, albeit after several years of hard work and revelations. He had transformed. Moreover, his firm recognized the change. He was asked to take on a larger, more significant leadership role, which not only resulted in his family relocating but his firm also made him financially whole after the consequences of his earlier behavioral difficulties.

Part of his new role involved mentoring, coaching, and sponsoring others—both those who had cresting leadership potential, as well as those who were encountering potholes in their careers. His intense personal journey became a rock-solid foundation for him to help others. The power of his pain and his success had forged into zeal. Formally, a real part of his job was to invest time and energy in others' success. Now, he could augment his skill with his own real tools, real stories, and the unique power that comes from living the journey. What had started from confusion and hard realities years before ended with growth and success for Tom both personally and professionally, transforming him as a leader. It was palpable.

During the final decade of his career, Tom sponsored over a dozen people into partnership at his firm. He became beloved as a coach and mentor. People who had originally reported in interviews how difficult he was, how self-important his affect was, now sought him out for advice and humility actually became part of his brand. Moreover, in the last two years before his retirement, he studied, engaged in a formal program, and became a certified executive coach himself. He plans to spend time during his retirement continuing his passion of coaching others.

Lesson 5: Propagation

What happens when someone who is coached elevates into a position of influence and their impact becomes exponential? That is John's story. Eight years ago, I got a call from a client asking if I would consider coaching a physician with whom they have a long-standing relationship. He had experienced a major physical change resulting from an accident that was life altering. He was physically, mentally, and spiritually challenged by that significant event. As would be expected with such a dramatic trauma, the event forged a dark night of the soul followed by epiphanies. Some presents come very poorly wrapped! Because the doctor emerged from a period of deep reflection and acceptance of his new physical realities, there were stirrings of new avenues where he could flex his professional muscles that would complement his existing practice of medicine. He is an exquisite surgeon and continues going forward accordingly, but as he grew he wanted to engage a coach to continue to make sense of how he was changing personally and professionally. Coaching was both about integrating new professional experiences and continuing to thrive within an already stellar career. As part of his refreshed trajectory, he wanted to create new opportunities to move young doctors forward in their medical acumen and especially in their leadership.

John's background lent itself to help in a big way. He was grounded in leadership development because he graduated from a renowned military service academy, rich in leadership education and tradition. His mentor was a luminary both in medicine and in extraordinary humanitarian service. In this new part of his new professional life, he was driven to very actively bring leadership education at medical schools to the fore. A compelling mission that required yeoman's work as well as nuanced competencies in fund raising, institutional politics, motivation, and structure to bring it all together. Coaching over the years has been squarely in the Transformational Growth category with occasional forays into the Total Engagement box of our model when it was called for to work through specific situational projects and opportunities.

The leadership program he spearheads is uniquely successful, having trained and graduated scores of medical professionals of all stripes—from students to interns to fellows. The program now also includes adjunct professionals such as physical therapists and nurses. They have all become stronger, more nuanced leaders due to their participation in the leadership program. The charge of these medical leaders is to bring new leadership "bones" to their home institutions and every future situation in which they work and lead, thus extending John's reach far beyond the practice of medicine. It is extending medical leadership into the future and into what we now know more viscerally than ever, is a changing, shifting world that needs the most effective doctors and the most effective leaders. Coaching has been part of John's ongoing journey to deliver on this mission.

HOW TO MAKE THE MOST OF EXECUTIVE COACHING

We hope that this exploration has piqued your interest in enlisting an executive coach to help you explore your potential and advance your career. As you begin your coaching journey here are our suggestions for how to maximize the experience:

- Expect the coach to help you reflect, not give you direction or advice. If you go into the relationship understanding that an executive coach's job is to support your own self-discovery you will walk out of the engagement with much more progress and satisfaction. Moreover, if you *really* want the coach's advice, ask for it! They may not give it to you, although often you will hear examples of what other coaching clients of theirs have done in similar situations, and sometimes that is all you need to help you come to your own decision about what you would like to try next.
- Data is key. Make sure your executive coach is going to help you gather some solid information that can give you insights into when and how you are at your best…and not. Assessments are not the only kind of data. You and your coach may decide to get more subjective information by having the coach engage in interviews about you. They will ask people you choose about what you do well, where the potholes you fall into are, what your brand is, how you work with teams, and what piece of unvarnished advice might be proffered.
- Finally, your mindset matters. If you are feeling coerced into a coaching relationship and frustrated about your situation, pause and ask yourself honestly about both what might be the source of your discomfort and what might be possible if coaching were successful for you. Courage is key. Being open to a coaching process performed by a relative stranger can be daunting. However, if you can turn your mindset into one that is willing to learn from the experience and exploration, you might be surprised about what you discover and where it takes you!

DISCLOSURE

The authors have nothing to disclose.

REFERENCES

1. Evered RD, Selman JC. Coaching and the art of management. Organ Dyn 1989; 18(2):16–32.

2. Albrecht K. Organization development: a total systems approach to positive change in any business organization. New Jersey: Prentice-Hall; 1983.
3. Grieves J. Strategic human resource development. London: Sage; 2003.
4. ICF 2020 Global Coaching Study: Executive Summary, 1–18.
5. Dyrbye LN, Shanafelt TD, Gill PR, et al. Effect of a professional coaching intervention on the well-being and distress of physicians: a pilot randomized clinical trial. JAMA Intern Med 2019;179(10):1406–14.
6. "When your Foundations Move, The Three Crucial Transitions in Life and Career" C. Michael Thompson, pg. 55
7. The Soul's Code: in search of character and calling, 6, 1996, Random House; New York, 135.
8. Lorsch JW, Tierney TJ. Aligning the Stars. In: PG, 21. Cambridge, MA: Harvard Business School Press; 2002.

Professional Coaching in Medicine and Health Care

Alyssa M. Stephany, MD, MS[a,b,c], Penny Archuleta, MA[d], Poonam Sharma, MD[e], Sharon K. Hull, MD, MPH[f],*

KEYWORDS

- Professional coaching • Coaching • Burnout • Provider well-being
- Organizational effectiveness • Leadership development • Career planning

KEY POINTS

- Professional coaching is a recognized modality for helping individuals and organizations develop skills that are important in health care.
- Coaching can impact four broad areas of health care: (1) the provider experience of working in health care, (2) role and career development, (3) team effectiveness, and (4) development of an organizational coaching culture.
- Much of the early development of the profession of coaching comes from the business world, and the modality has gained traction, and evidence to support its use in health care in recent years.
- Professional coaching is a healing modality that can benefit health care providers, their patients, their families and other key stakeholders, and the organizations in which they work.

INTRODUCTION

Health care and coaching, although two separate professions, are somewhat similar in that they both seek to gather information and provide solutions or insights through the process of asking questions. Like health care, coaching is a broad and diverse industry. Contemporary understanding of coaching is predicated on the concept that the process of asking questions on the part of the coach elicits insight in the individual, group or team being coached. Some common definitions of coaching are:

[a] Leadership Center for Physicians, Children's Mercy Kansas City, 2401 Gillham Road, Kansas City, MO 64108, USA; [b] University of Missouri, Kansas City School of Medicine; [c] University of Kansas School of Medicine; [d] Department of Medicine, University of Colorado and Children's Hospital Colorado, 12631 East 17th Avenue, Mail Stop B178, Aurora, CO 80045, USA; [e] Department of Pathology, Creighton University School of Medicine, CHI Health, 13659 Cuming Street, Omaha, NE 68154, USA; [f] Department of Family Medicine, University of North Carolina at Chapel Hill School of Medicine and Metta Solutions, LLC, 3307 Watkins Road, Suite 159, Durham, NC 27707, USA
* Corresponding author.
E-mail address: Sharon.hull@mettasolutions.com

Clin Sports Med 42 (2023) 195–208
https://doi.org/10.1016/j.csm.2022.11.001
0278-5919/23/© 2022 Elsevier Inc. All rights reserved.

sportsmed.theclinics.com

- Coaching involves unlocking people's potential to maximize their own performance.[1]
- Coaching is the process of helping people discover and use tools, knowledge, and opportunities they need to develop themselves and become more effective.[2]
- Coaching is partnering with clients in a thought-provoking and creative process that inspires them to maximize their personal and professional potential.[3]

Although coaching, mentoring and therapy have some things in common, they are distinct professional activities and the intellectual framework for each approach is different.

Coaching uses a process of inquiry and personal discovery to build the coachee's level of awareness and provides them with a structured process of exploration support, and feedback. A coach guides the client on the path of self-knowledge and skill building, providing accountability along the way.

Mentoring occurs when someone with personal and professional expertise shares their experience and offers advice to someone with less experience, so they have a deeper insight into the issues and challenges they are facing.[4] The mentee may or may not choose to follow the mentor's guidance. A mentor can be seen as a wise and trusted counselor, teacher, or adviser.

The differences between coaching and psychotherapy are vast.[5] Therapy is often focused on the assessment and treatment of pathology based on events in the past, whereas coaching is a future-focused and insight-oriented approach that intends to enhance normal functioning. In psychotherapy, the therapist is an expert. In coaching, the coachee, rather than the coach, is the expert for their own life. Unlike the practice of psychotherapy, mentoring and coaching are not regulated by state or federal licensure in the United States, though coaching is a regulated profession in many other countries. Coaching professionals do not diagnose, nor do they offer therapeutic treatment or intervention.

Within the past 20 years, professional organizations such as the International Coach Federation,[3] EMCC Global[6] and the International Association of Coaching[7] have created standards to help guide the practice. Professional coaches receive certification through training programs accredited through these or other accrediting bodies. In this article, we use the term professional coaching to delineate services provided by someone who has formal training and credentialing in coaching methodology and ethics. There is great value in teaching coaching skills to nonprofessional coaches, and in using peer coaching to enhance coaching skills and peer support in an organization. We believe that these are separate and distinct functions when compared with professional coaching.

BACKGROUND: EMERGING PERSPECTIVE ON THE USE OF COACHING IN HEALTH CARE

Historically, coaching aimed at remediation has been used in health care for struggling providers and learners who fail to meet expectations and thus need to significantly improve their job performance or face the possibility of dismissal. Over time, coaching has come to be viewed more proactively as an investment in talent for which a return on the investment is expected in terms of measurable benchmarks. This transition has happened in part because of the outcomes that have been demonstrated in nonpunitive settings. The literature around coaching effectiveness has shown its benefit as a developmental tool.

The health care sector has begun to embrace coaching to promote resilience and innovation during a time of massive disruption while also cultivating healthier workplace cultures. The prevalence of burnout symptoms among physicians is high, with those at the front lines of care at especially high risk.[8] Symptoms of burnout are nearly twice as common among physicians than among US workers in other fields.[9] The coronavirus disease-2019 (COVID-19) pandemic has added another layer of risk to the already overwhelmed workforce. Physician burnout and fatigue are independently associated with major medical errors.[10] Professional coaching has proven to be an effective way to reduce emotional exhaustion and burnout as well as improve performance, retention, quality of life, and resilience for physicians.[9,11] In 2008, Cleveland Clinic instituted a peer-based coaching and mentoring program for physicians to promote a proactive approach to clinician well-being, which has reportedly saved the health system at least $133 million in physician retention.[12] In addition to retention, physicians in this program experienced an increased sense of accomplishment, purpose, and engagement.

Box 1 describes the core competencies a professional coach should show to be effective in their work. Professional coaching works by "establishing a helping relationship with a developmental focus played out in conversations that stimulate the person or group being coached to greater awareness, deeper and broader thought, and wiser decisions and actions."[14] Coaching can be focused on individuals or on teams or groups, with a focus on different coaching skill sets applied in each of these settings.

COACHING AND THE CURRENT HEALTH CARE ENVIRONMENT

Rapid change, unprecedented growth in medical knowledge and technologies, staffing shortages, high turnover, political and economic uncertainty, competing obligations in professional and personal life, the trend toward increasing patient volumes, and the ongoing aftermath of a global pandemic[15] all combine to ensure health care organizations and the health care workforce are under constant pressure. Demands of the environment require systems, organizations, teams, and individuals who collaborate effectively, develop and work in functional teams, focus on service, establish mutual accountability and respect, deliver patient-centered care and leverage technology to gain efficiencies.[16,17]

These characteristics create tensions within the historically hierarchical and expert-centered model of medicine. Today's health care environment requires intentional transformation of this model to a new one that embraces and leverages more humane

---

Box 1
Core competencies to be expected of professional coaches[13]

Shows ethical practice

Embodies a coaching mindset—open, curious, flexible, and client-centered

Establishes and maintains agreements in partnership with the client and relevant stakeholders

Cultivates trust and safety

Maintains full presence with the client

Listens actively

Facilitates client awareness and insight

Facilitates client transformation and growth

and sustainable modes of work. One way to support individuals and organizations in effectively creating a new model of work in health care is by providing coaching, a profession whose very nature lies in personal and organizational development through support for change.[18,19]

An International Coaching Federation (ICF) Global Coach Client Survey ($N = 2130$)[20] indicated that regardless of type of engagement or primary objectives, most clients experience a benefit in areas directly related to the needs of health care providers. **Table 1** provides a list of potential areas where coaching could provide high-impact success for individual health care providers and organizations.

There are four broad areas of health care where we believe that professional coaching can have the most significant impact. These are (1) the provider experience of working in health care, (2) role and career development, (3) team effectiveness, and (4) development of an organizational coaching culture.

PROVIDER EXPERIENCE OF WORKING IN HEALTH CARE

Adapted from the Institute for Healthcare Improvement's 2008 Triple Aim framework for optimizing health system performance reflecting the key aims of enhancing patient experience, improving population health, and reducing cost, the 2014 proposed Quadruple Aim expanded the model to include and emphasize provider wellness as a key contributor to achieving true optimization of health care and associated outcomes. The addition of the fourth aim has been widely accepted and its importance recognized as organizations develop increased understanding of the prevalence and impact of provider burnout on multiple aspects of care.[21,22]

Burnout, dissatisfaction, and lack of engagement contribute to the shortage of practicing doctors and nurses as seen in the number of physicians leaving the profession, high nursing turnover, and increased physician suicide rates. Although external and internal pressures remain, coaching can help individuals focus on and build core skills that support resilience. Coaching can help individuals set realistic goals and develop

Table 1 Areas for potential high-impact change in health care organizations as a result of professional coaching[20]	
At the individual level	Interpersonal relationship skills Communication skills Work performance and efficiency Time management Career strategies Work/life alignment or balance Human well-being and resilience Perspective taking Imposter phenomenon Personal accountability Development of a service orientation Development of a learning and growth mindset Individual-level support in times of stress, duress or trauma
At the organizational level	Leadership skills Organizational perspective taking Stakeholder engagement Employee engagement and retention Team effectiveness Development of a positive organizational culture Organization-level support in times of stress, duress or trauma

action plans, enhance communication and problem-solving skills, build self-awareness and self-regulation skills, enhancing areas deemed key for resilience: connection, wellness, healthy thinking and meaning.[23]

Specific to health care providers, as depicted in the National Academy of Medicine's conceptual model for Clinician Well-Being and Resilience, provider wellness is multi-factorial.[24] Clinician well-being, clinician-patient relationships and ultimately patient well-being are affected by external pressures as well as internal factors, skills, and abilities. With increased pressures, physician burnout continues to increase. This trend is expected to continue as impact of the COVID-19 pandemic on provider resilience and well-being is assessed.[25]

By "partnering with clients in a thought-provoking and creative process that inspires them to maximize their personal and professional potential,"[3] a professional coach can help the client or team create positive learning and work environments. Such environments enable a shift in attention, enhanced meaning and purpose in work, alignment of values and expectations, job control, flexibility and autonomy, professional relationships, social support, work–life integration, and healthy organizational culture. These environmental qualities are integral contributing factors that support provider wellness and resilience. Such an environment can enhance retention of critical staff[12,26] while supporting individual well-being.

A coach may also be engaged for support when duress, stress or distress occurs. Increased societal awareness of the challenging nature of health care demands and the individual and collective impact of increased compassion fatigue, moral injury, burnout and disengagement among a wide range of health care professionals has enhanced awareness of the potential benefit of professional coaching to support attentiveness to well-being and reinforce resilience practices. A coach may also prove to have a positive impact in support for exploring and rediscovering joy among individual providers.[27]

In the wake of the COVID-19 pandemic response virtual coaching and technology-driven coaching companies such as BetterUp, Torch and others have experienced exponential growth in demand due to scalability of virtual services and reporting of positive outcomes.[28] Similar niche programs designed for scalability continue to develop with success. An example of this concept can be seen in a recently published article reflecting positive outcomes for a 6-month online, group coaching program designed to increase self-compassion, reduce burnout, moral injury and Imposter syndrome among female resident physicians. This intervention resulted in statistically significant reduction in the emotional exhaustion subscale of burnout compared with the control group.[29]

It is critical that coaches and clients understand that, when coaching in situations of duress, stress or distress, coaches must be attentive to use of appropriate coach competencies[13] in the delivery of coaching and not engage in psychotherapy. Although similar in nature, therapy lies in the realm of a licensed therapist. Coaches must be readily able to discern when the client needs acute or long-term mental health care and refer appropriately. Attention to the differences and boundaries for each profession is critical to the ethical practice of professional coaching.

ROLE AND CAREER DEVELOPMENT

The importance of leadership and role development has taken on new meaning and importance as turnover and staffing shortages in health care organizations trend up, impact from the pandemic continues and organizations establish initiatives to support workforce stability. Coach engagements and the support they provide may align with the need to support those promoted to leadership roles or given expanded scope and responsibility. This is particularly true in a time of extreme uncertainty and stress, for people with limited training or prior experience in leadership and for those the organization is looking to retain, retrain or develop.[30–32]

A coach may be engaged at a variety of times in a client's career, specifically during key role transitions and shifts into new levels of leadership. Such role-based coaching provides support for those shifting from the role of an individual contributor to a leader or to a leader of leaders. Health care professional training is almost exclusively focused on the provider's clinical skill set and provides very little, if any, training about leadership. Providers are often promoted into leadership positions or seek such positions with a belief (on their part and that of others) that their clinical expertise and success will naturally translate to effectiveness and success in leadership. This is not always a sound assumption, and many health care providers benefit from specific attention to the development of core leadership skills. A coach can provide opportunity for reflection, establishing an action plan to identify areas for development and enhance effectiveness of these skills.[33]

TEAM EFFECTIVENESS

Team coaching within organizations is a growing field of practice and research. The process and goals of team coaching vary, with ICF perhaps having the clearest definition of this professional coaching specialty. Team Coaching is defined by ICF as "partnering in a co-creative and reflective process with a team on its dynamics and relationships in a way that inspires them to maximize their abilities and potential to reach their common purpose and shared goals."[34]

Team coaching may be an independent engagement but is often used in tandem with the coaching of an individual or individuals on the team so that efforts and desired outcomes can be synthesized. It may overlay or be used in conjunction with other aspects of team development such as team building or team training. Team coaching is often longer in duration than individual coaching, allowing for more in-depth exploration of team characteristics, alignment and achievement of goals and support for sustainable practices.[35]

A review of the Agency for Healthcare Research and Quality (AHRQ) Safety Program for Ambulatory Surgery provides an example of team coaching designed to enhance patient care and positively impact team communications. The coaching process begins with an observation, feedback from the coach to the team, and the posing of open-ended questions to support the team in finding their own solutions and best practices. Effective communication skills such as approaching the client from a stance of curiosity, reflecting back or mirroring the client's or teams statements, and other active listening skills are modeled for the team by the coach.[36]

DEVELOPING AN ORGANIZATIONAL CULTURE OF COACHING

System-level coaching can be offered in targeted areas but may be best deployed in the service of building a healthy organizational culture. To maximize impact and improve the success of system-level coaching engagements, it is recommended that organizations consider ways to develop a culture of coaching and infuse this culture into system-wide organizational processes including:

- Talent development
- Performance feedback
- Communication skills

- Strategic career management
- Team development
- Remediation, activation of feedback, and improved performance

Coaching cultures exist when an organization identifies and embraces a coaching approach as a key aspect of its leadership and development strategy. A culture that embraces coaching supports and empowers its individuals, teams, and leaders in a process of learning and growth. Leaders, managers, and employees use coaching skills and techniques to create a supportive high-performance environment and external coaches are leveraged when needed.

Organizations with coaching cultures create and sustain psychological safety, which in turn helps with employee retention, improves productivity and performance, and positively impacts employee wellness. In a study of a high-impact talent management process[37] system-wide deployment of professional coaching was found to be the talent process with the greatest overall positive business impact.

Coaching may support several components of talent development, including.

- Accelerated learning with high potential through a longitudinal coach engagement
- Integration of leadership development program concepts and content through participant coaching
- Commitment to all new leaders for a six-month coach engagement to support onboarding
- Transitions to new roles
- Remediation coaching for targeted behavior change.

Communication skill development can be accelerated through work with a coach. Through communication style assessments and the coaching practice of asking powerful questions, a coach can help a client or team identify areas of challenge in communication with others. As the client or clients gain awareness of their foundational communication strengths and their areas for development, the two can work together to co-create a path for skill building. Specific communication skills to be addressed might include the ability to vary messages to different target audience, making effective public presentations, crisis communications, conflict management and providing effective feedback.

Building communication skills within the system might also be achieved through multiple interventions that a coach might be involved in or aligned with for reinforcement. An example of this might be a system seeking to develop effective communication skills within their workforce. Competencies to build might include active listening, direct communication and conflict management. A plan might include selection and application of a common multi-rater (360) assessment with coach debrief for leaders to identify strengths and challenges in context of communication, real-time virtual or in-person workshops or an asynchronous course on active listening skills. This type of multi-faceted intervention supports skill building and sustainability of newly acquired skills across many individuals in ways that support the deep development of a coaching culture.

A note about the patient experience of care and patient outcomes

The patient experience of care and patient outcomes are inextricably related to the provider experience of working in health care. Examples such as the Agency for Healthcare Research and Quality (AHRQ) program noted above[36] illustrate how coaching of individuals and teams in health care organizations and development of a coaching culture can have both direct and indirect impact on the interactions of providers with their colleagues, patients, and team members.

Coaching has shown to be an effective method for enhanced provider well-being, which correlates with safe and effective patient care[38] Quality and patient safety is jeopardized by provider distress, staff turnover, team morale, and decreased cohesiveness of the whole health care enterprise.[9] The potential benefits of professional coaching and of creating a coaching culture in organizations can serve to enhance the ultimate bottom line of health care, the experience of the patient who is seeking care, and the patient's maximal safety and best possible outcomes.

CASE STUDIES IN THE USE OF PROFESSIONAL COACHING ACROSS THE LIFE COURSE OF A CAREER

The success of coaching depends on meeting the coachee's needs, in a similar way that effective health care depends on meeting a patient's needs. Coaching addresses issues across the lifespan of a career, whether at the beginning or end of an individual's career, when they are facing personal or professional challenges, or when challenges occur that impact personal and professional life at the same time. Coaching allows individuals to address various challenges and intentionally consider the whole person, no matter the challenges they face.

Topics such as burnout, career decisions, evolving one's mindset, and crafting enduring legacies can manifest at any point during a career for any health care professional without predictability or linearity. We include case scenarios here which are composites of many academic health care professionals who have been part of the authors' coaching experiences engaging with professional leadership coaches in academic institutions. These scenarios will allow the reader to sample the potential types of situations in which coaching can be helpful. The case scenarios below do not reflect nor are they intended to represent any one identifiable individual.

Early Career Case Scenario: Burnout

Coachee A, an assistant professor and advanced practice provider, was four years into an emergency medicine career when he began to examine his career choices. He questioned his purpose, if he would ever feel joy in work and his desires for the future. Instead of being enthusiastic about his work, he felt only an unending tunnel of misery stretched in front of him. Although his leader was mentoring him, he felt directionless and uninterested in the aspects of his career that initially motivated and excited him about pursuing a career as a health care provider. He was despondent. His leader recommended coaching to help him find insight and meaningful goals for himself.

When the faculty member began coaching, he expressed feeling overwhelmed by work and out of balance. He could not remember the last time he wanted to engage with patients. The coach strongly recommended that the provider seek an initial mental health evaluation to delineate any issues that needed to be addressed on that front, in tandem with professional coaching, and the provider did seek this additional care. Once mental health issues were addressed, the coaching engagement focused on the barriers to successfully completing just one work shift at a time. These barriers ranged from challenges arising from use of the electronic health record, constant policy and protocol changes related to the COVID-19 pandemic response, staff and employee shortages, personal safety concerns, and the burden out of discharging patients without adequate resources. He described himself as burned out and feeling so exhausted that he just wanted to walk away from it all.

For many weeks, he explored his feelings of being traumatized, the influence of his medical work and service to patients, and strategies to feel more empowered in those situations. To combat these negative feelings, he focused on self-care and evaluating his activities to remove those overextending his bandwidth. He noted small, good things that happened in his days, took opportunities to find joy in patient encounters, reframed his perspective on his work and explored his sphere of control. In addition, he brainstormed strategies to feel more empowered to navigate the barriers he encountered rather than helpless in the face of them. In the three months following his initial exploration, the provider reported decreased burnout, increased engagement, and the ability to actively reframe challenges from a critical lens to a more solution-focused lens.

Mid-Career Case Scenario: Deciding About a New Opportunity

Fifteen years into a career as a specialty physician, Coachee B, an associate professor, received an invitation to interview for an institutional leadership position. This person had achieved national excellence in the clinical realm, had recognized expertise in quality improvement and quality assessment, was productive in terms of scholarly activity, and was widely recognized as a successful clinical and administrative leader. Despite her achievements, she experienced periods of self-doubt, feelings of inadequacy, and moments of comparing herself to her peers. When she entered a professional coaching engagement, she was a medical director, fellowship director, clinician, and active researcher. Applying for this new position posed a job opportunity representing a fork in the road. If she took the job, she would need to step out of some of the roles that still held interest for her and move toward a new professional space where she would have a steep learning curve.

Through coaching and the use of techniques such as visualization exercises, she found insights within herself. She discovered that she often sabotaged the opportunities presented to her, both consciously and unconsciously. She identified a specific fear of change and the unknown regarding the opportunity in front of her. She realized the aspects of herself that she would have to adapt to face the discomfort and uncertainty. She could decide on the job opportunity by re-examining her values, assessing her strengths, challenging beliefs that were not necessarily her own, and evaluating her career overall. In working to increase confidence in her choice, she uncovered a concept that was new to her—no decision or career choice must be permanent. She learned that one can decide to pivot if new data or information comes to light. Ultimately, she described feeling empowered enough by this introspection to reach a decision that felt authentic and realistic with a high probability of success.

Senior Career Case Scenario: Evolution of Career Toward Developing and Promoting Others

A physician and full professor of surgery, Coachee C, was well-respected as a surgeon and as a senior faculty member who had dedicated his career to improving care delivery for a particular patient population. As a continual lifelong learner, he initially engaged with a professional coach to achieve what he referred to as work–life integration. He also sought insights on developing life habits that would forward his career goals.

He had reached a point in his career where he had fulfilled most of his professional goals. As a result, he grappled with shifting from setting and achieving practical goals to not having an ongoing project and feeling empty and as though there might be nothing left to for him to accomplish. He wanted insight into what meaning he needed to create in the later part of his career and what mindset he desired to develop for this career phase. He wanted the ability to apply his talents and strengths and longed to feel still challenged and inspired with his work. He no longer felt that more accomplishments would give him what he sought. Through coaching, he did purposeful work to discover what he enjoyed doing. In the process of inquiry-based coaching, he was challenged to reflect on powerful questions asked by his coach and found that he wanted to evolve into more than just a mentor and a consultant to more junior faculty. He wanted to help them uncover insights, foster a growth mindset, and develop into the next generation of leaders, educators, researchers, and clinicians, who advance the overall mission of medicine. He pursued career development to evolve into a faculty member who empowers others to seek their insights and develop their dreams into reality. As a result, he crafted an authentic venue for people to share their experiences about their careers in ways participants felt allowed them to be true to themselves. After over ten months, he realized his career fulfillment came from a different perch within the institutional structure, thus expanding his reach from personal career impact with direct patient care to a more widespread career impact mentoring the next generation.

Capstone Case Scenario: Legacy and Purpose

Coachee D, a full professor nearing retirement, with a notable career in her specialty as a clinician scientist and a leader, wanted to discover what the next step was for her in the penultimate stages of her career. She was uncertain whether she wanted to pursue full retirement, phased retirement, or perhaps redefine herself with an encore career. By completing a values exercise with her coach, she gained clarity about her values, and how they related to her desire to create a legacy.

Notably, though, she was unclear about what pathway would lead her to feel settled with this capstone portion of her career in medicine. She desired purpose and meaning in the upcoming phase of her career, yet she knew she would be unable to continue at the current pace or time and energy investment that she was giving to her career. During her years in medicine, she had a wide range of experiences as a consultant, a community mentor for high schoolers interested in the sciences and as an innovator on a medical society foundation. She had other experiences beyond her professional interests that had expanded her concept of her whole self in theater, art, and music. She was intrigued by these interests as she explored how she wanted to spend her time. A large central part of her every day was filled with mental and emotional energy dedicated to medicine. Knowing this, she anticipated a grieving process and understood that she would need to adapt. She was uncertain how to do this.

Through a professional coaching engagement, she wanted to explore how to remain authentic and explore what she desired as the next step in her life journey. In her work with her coach, she challenged her current perceptions of what her day-to-day job could be, and what that work would be if it aligned with her values. She decided that she was ready for retirement from most of her clinical and research activities. As she worked with her coach about the uncertainty of what lay ahead, she found a way to truly celebrate and honor where she had been, what she had accomplished, yet eagerly explore what was the next stage for herself. She decided to stay on the medical staff as a non-admitting member, that she would dedicate herself to the efforts of diversity, equity, and inclusion as the institution developed and built the infrastructure for a role of a medical director in that space, and that she would eventually investigate what Professor Emerita status might look like for her when she was ready.

Outside of the institution's walls, she was able to represent her profession by helping establish a more formal program for high schoolers to grow awareness of medical careers. She also found a way to further develop her artistic skills and used them to create paintings that celebrated the various parts of her career. Although this understanding of her goals and the meaning she wanted to make of her life would continue to develop, she felt she had grown in a way that would allow her to reassess where she was every year and what she wanted her career to look like in the year ahead, staying true to her known purpose and the meaning of her journey.

These case scenarios are representative of the many ways in which professional coaching can be helpful to professionals in the health care arena. Other common coaching topics include navigating institutional politics, navigating very real structural discrimination for minorities, women and others who are sometimes marginalized in health care institutions, development of effective communication skills, and time management. All these topics are common challenges for health care professionals and are highly amenable to work with a professional coach.

DISCUSSION

As we have shown in this review of the nature of coaching in health care, the evidence supporting its use and case scenarios that offer examples of its deployment, professional coaching can address several institutional and individual issues. For the individual, professional and peer coaching have been shown to help reduce burnout and to improve job satisfaction, improving the overall provider experience of health care. Coaching is also beneficial for and can be a critical factor in successful role and career development. It is a modality that may be particularly beneficial as the world, and western society in general, emerge from the current global pandemic and its impact on health care and the related shifts in perceptions of the nature of the daily work of health care professionals.

For institutions and teams that work within them, there is evidence to support the effectiveness of professional and peer coaching in improving team function, managing change and understanding leadership roles. It can also enhance team effectiveness and can benefit the overall organization through development of a systemic coaching culture. With the cost of turnover estimated to be up to three times an employee's annual salary, investment in an institution-wide coaching program Is worth the investment in terms of reducing losses from employee turnover.[12]

Professional coaching can help human beings in a very challenging profession make sense and meaning of the challenges they face, discover their best approach to meeting those challenges, and make good choices about their professional and personal lives. It can help them discover (or rediscover) their authentic self and find ways to align their own goals and values to the demands of the profession. This is a healing process that occurs over the course of a professional lifetime.

For health care providers, their patients, their learners, their families and other stakeholders whose lives they impact, use of this ongoing healing modality can make a tremendous difference in the experience of the provider and stakeholders in being fully human while still being fully professional.

For health care organizations, this supportive investment in the well-being of highly talented individuals is not just a bottom-line concern, though it does and can significantly affect costs associated with professional turnover, burnout and errors in health care. It is also a supremely important way in which organizations can show the value they place on the human beings who do the work of patient care, research, teaching and leadership in those organizations.

SUMMARY

We have shown in this article some of the evidence supporting the use of professional coaching in health care, some practical applications of this healing modality in the lives of individuals, and a framework from which to consider this work.

Organizations can show significant commitment to provider well-being by developing and using robust and systematic professional coaching programs (either internal to or external to the organization) to support individuals, teams, emerging leaders and the overall system. Doing so can be a significant boon to all who are impacted by the health care system.

DISCLOSURE

S.K. Hull has no commercial or financial conflicts of interest or funding sources to disclose. She owns and directs a professional executive coaching and consulting company, Metta Solutions, LLC, which provides professional executive coaching and consulting services. P. Sharma has no financial conflict of interest or funding sources to disclose. She owns Sharma Healthcare Coaching and Consulting, LLC, which provides executive coaching services. P. Archuleta has no commercial or financial conflicts of interest or funding sources to disclose. A.M. Stephany has no commercial or financial conflicts of interest or funding sources to disclose.

REFERENCES

1. Whitmore J. Coaching for performance: the principles and practice of coaching and leadership. 5th Edition (Updated 25th Anniversary Edition. London: Nicholas Brealey; 2017.
2. Peterson DB, Hicks MD. Leader as coach: strategies for coaching and developing others. Minneapolis: Personnel Decisions International Corporation; 1996.
3. International Coaching Federation. About ICF. International Coach Federation. Available at: https://coachfederation.org/about#:~:text=ICF%20defines%20coaching%20as%20partnering,their%20personal%20and%20professional%20potential. Accessed August 5, 2022.
4. Kram KE. Mentoring at work: developmental relationships in organizational life. Glenview, IL: Scott Foresman and Company; 1985.
5. Westfall C. Battling Burnout, Anxiety And Building Productivity: Do You Need Coaching Or Therapy? Forbes. Available at: https://www.forbes.com/sites/chriswestfall/2021/08/25/battling-burnout-anxiety-and-building-productivity-do-you-need-coaching-or-therapy/. Accessed August 22, 2022.
6. EMCC Global. EMCC Global. 2022. Available at: https://www.emccglobal.org/. Accessed August 13, 2022.
7. International Association of Coaching. Home - International Association of Coaching. @IACcoachmastery. 2022. Available at: https://certifiedcoach.org/. Accessed August 13, 2022.
8. Shanafelt TD, West CP, Sinsky C, et al. Changes in Burnout and Satisfaction With Work–life Integration in Physicians and the General US Working Population Between 2011 and 2017. Mayo Clin Proc 2019;94(9):1681–94.
9. Gazelle G, Liebschutz JM, Riess H. Physician burnout: coaching a way out. J Gen Intern Med 2015;30(4):508–13.
10. Tawfik DS, Profit J, Morgenthaler TI, et al. Physician Burnout, Well-being, and Work Unit Safety Grades in Relationship to Reported Medical Errors. Mayo Clin Proc 2018;93(11):1571–80.

11. Dyrbye LN, Shanafelt TD, Gill PR, et al. Effect of a Professional Coaching Intervention on the Well-being and Distress of Physicians. JAMA Intern Med 2019; 179(10):1406.

12. Gleeson C., How Cleveland Clinic has saved $133M in physician retention, *Becker's Hosp Rev*, 2022. Available at: https://www.beckershospitalreview.com/hospital-physician-relationships/how-cleveland-clinic-has-saved-133m-in-physician-retention.html. Accessed November 23, 2021.

13. International Coaching Federation. The Gold Standard in Coaching | ICF - Core Competencies. 2022. Available at: https://coachingfederation.org/credentials-and-standards/core-competencies. Accessed August 10, 2022.

14. Riddle DD, Hoole ER, Gullette ECD. In: *The Center for Creative Leadership Handbook of Coaching in Organizations*. San Francisco, CA: Jossey-Bass; 2015.

15. Shreffler J, Huecker M, Petrey J. The Impact of COVID-19 on Healthcare Worker Wellness: A Scoping Review. West J Emerg Med 2020;21(5). https://doi.org/10.5811/westjem.2020.7.48684.

16. Enders T. and Conroy J., Advancing the Academic Health System for the Future, Future of Academic Medicine Series, Association of American Medical Colleges Available at: https://store.aamc.org/advancing-the-academic-health-system-for-the-future-pdf.html, 2014. Accessed December 17, 2022.

17. Johnson K.V., Boston-Fleschhauer C. and Duke-Mosier S., Staff turnover: 4 key takeaways from Advisory Board's survey of 224 hospitals, Daily Briefing Available at: https://www.advisory.com/Daily-Briefing/2022/03/09/hospital-turnover-survey, 2022. Accessed December 17, 2022.

18. Winters R., Coaching Physicians to become leaders, *Harv Business Rev*, 2013. Available at: https://hbr.org/2013/10/coaching-physicians-to-become-leaders. Accessed October 7, 2013. Accessed December 17, 2022.

19. Qadir X.C., Kassauei K., Norz B., et al., The Healthcare Industry: ready For Coaching? 2020. 11/17/2020, Available at: https://instituteofcoaching.org/blogs/healthcare-industry-ready-coaching. Accessed December 17, 2022.

20. Association Resource Centre Incorporated, PricewaterhouseCoopers LLP. ICF Global Coaching Client Study (Executive Summary. 2009. Available at: https://researchportal.coachfederation.org/Document/Pdf/abstract_190.

21. Berwick DM, Nolan TW, Whittington J. The Triple Aim: Care, Health, And Cost. Health Aff 2008;27(3):759–69.

22. Bodenheimer T, Sinsky C. From Triple to Quadruple Aim: Care of the Patient Requires Care of the Provider. The Ann Fam Med 2014;12(6):573–6.

23. Building your resilience. American Psychological Association. Available at: https://www.apa.org/topics/resilience/building-your-resilience. Accessed August 29, 2022.

24. Medcine NAo. Factors Affecting Clinician Well-Being and Resilience - Conceptual Model. 2018. Clinician Well-Being Knowledge Hub Available at: https://nam.edu/clinicianwellbeing/resources/factors-affecting-clinician-well-being-and-resilience-conceptual-model/?_sf_s=conceptual+model.

25. National Academy of Medicine. Action collaborative on clinician well-being and resilience: program description. National Academy of Medicine. Available at: https://nam.edu/initiatives/clinician-resilience-and-well-being/. Accessed August 22, 2022.

26. Cohn KH, Bethancourt B, Simington M. The Lifelong Iterative Process of Physician Retention - ProQuest. J Healthc Manag 2009;54(4):220–6.

27. Newton R. Rediscover Joy at Work. Harvard Business Review. 2021. Available at https://hbr.org/2021/09/rediscover-joy-at-work. Accessed December 17, 2022.

28. Bersin J. Online Coaching Is So Hot It's Now Disrupting Leadership Development. Insights on Corporate Talent, Learning and HR Technology blog. 2022. Available at: https://joshbersin.com/2022/01/online-coaching-is-so-hot-its-now-disrupting-leadership-development/.

29. Fainstad T, Mann A, Suresh K, et al. Effect of a Novel Online Group-Coaching Program to Reduce Burnout in Female Resident Physicians. JAMA Netw Open 2022; 5(5):e2210752.

30. Cable S, Graham E. Leading Better Care": An evaluation of an accelerated coaching intervention for clinical nursing leadership development. J Nurs Manag 2018;26(5):605–12.

31. Shanafelt T, Trockel M, Rodriguez A, et al. Wellness-Centered Leadership: Equipping Health Care Leaders to Cultivate Physician well-Being and Professional Fulfillment. Acad Med 2021;96(5):641–51.

32. Shanafelt TD, Gorringe G, Menaker R, et al. Impact of organizational leadership on physician burnout and satisfaction. Mayo Clin Proc 2015;90(4):432–40.

33. Lee TH. Turning Doctors into Leaders. Harvard Business Review. 2010;(2010). Available at: https://hbr.org/2010/04/turning-doctors-into-leaders. Accessed December 17, 2022.

34. International Coaching Federation. Team Coaching Competencies - International Coaching Federation. 2022. Available at: https://coachingfederation.org/team-coaching-competencies. Accessed August 10, 2022.

35. Cassatly MG, Bergquist WH. The Broken Covenant in U.S. Healthcare - ProQuest. J Med Pract Manage 2022;(3):136–9.

36. Agency for Healthcare Research and Quality. TeamSTEPPS 2.0: Module 9. Coaching Workshop. 2022. Available at: https://www.ahrq.gov/teamstepps/instructor/fundamentals/module9/igcoaching.html. Accessed August 10, 2022.

37. Bersin J. Coaching: An Imperative for Leaders. Insights on Corporate Talent, Learning and HR Technology blog. 2007. Available at: https://joshbersin.com/2007/06/coaching-an-imperative-for-leaders/.

38. Dyrbye LN, Shanafelt TD, Gill PR, et al. Effect of a professional coaching intervention on the well-being and distress of physicians: a pilot randomized clinical trial. JAMA Intern Med 2019;179(10):1406–14.

Coaching for the Orthopedic Surgery Leader

David N. Bernstein, MD, MBA, MEI[a], Kevin J. Bozic, MD, MBA[b],*

KEYWORDS

- Coaching • Orthopedic surgery leaders • Health-care delivery • Burnout • Coachee
- Leadership • Professional development

KEY POINTS

- Orthopedic surgery leaders have countless professional and personal responsibilities, which can become overwhelming at times; coaching can assist in optimizing efficiency and outcomes.
- Coaching can assist in addressing burnout, optimizing performance, and inspiring orthopedic surgery leaders to continue to push themselves to improve every day.
- With the level of expertise, technical skills, and passion needed to excel, orthopedic surgeons share many of the qualities that high-level athletes and musicians possess; thus, coaching can help orthopedic surgeons achieve their full potential.
- Coaching can be either individual-based through a professional coach or peer-to-peer, with both providing different benefits and learning opportunities.
- The value of coaching for orthopedic surgery leaders should not be underestimated.

INTRODUCTION

From the increase in telehealth to the expansion of private investors to the growth of transparency (both price and patient outcomes) and value-based care initiatives, health-care delivery is rapidly changing in the United States and globally.[1] With this evolution of health-care delivery, leaders across the health-care sector—including within orthopedic surgery—have needed to rapidly adapt to the changing landscape to optimize value delivered to patients. Demand for musculoskeletal care continues to rapidly increase, with more than 1.7 billion people globally suffering from musculoskeletal conditions.[2] At the same time, workforce challenges have caused substantial issues, especially since the onset of the coronavirus disease 2019 global pandemic.[3] In addition, personal responsibilities (eg, family and other personal commitments) remain, and, in many instances, are delayed or even sacrificed because of the constant onslaught of professional responsibilities from being a health-care professional.

[a] Harvard Combined Orthopaedic Residency Program, Massachusetts General Hospital, 55 Fruit Street, Boston, MA 02114 USA; [b] Department of Surgery and Perioperative Care, Dell Medical School at The University of Texas at Austin, 1701 Trinity Street, Austin, TX 78712, USA
* Corresponding author.
E-mail address: kevin.bozic@austin.utexas.edu

Clin Sports Med 42 (2023) 209–217
https://doi.org/10.1016/j.csm.2022.12.002
0278-5919/23/Published by Elsevier Inc.

sportsmed.theclinics.com

When considered together, these factors have a major impact on the health-care de-livery environment and pose enormous challenges and increased stressors on ortho-pedic surgeons and their teams.

One of the more negative outcomes of these many changing and "moving parts" for orthopedic surgeons today is burnout. A recent study found about 38% of all physi-cians' specialties had at least one or more symptoms of burnout,[4] which is at or slightly less than the level orthopedic surgeons report symptoms of burnout.[5] Not only does burnout affect an orthopedic surgeon's professional well-being but also it can have dire personal ramification.[6] Further, there are ongoing scholarly endeavors to better understand how burnout may negatively affect patient clinical outcomes as well, although more research is needed in this area.[7] Tackling physician burnout is central to optimizing a health-care delivery system that delivers high value care, including musculoskeletal care.

Beyond burnout, ever-increasing administrative tasks paired with policy changes that place increased burden on physicians and decrease reimbursement without appropriate risk-adjustment have been central challenges facing orthopedic surgery leaders. For example, prior authorization continues to negatively influence clinical practice,[8] taking away from direct patient care. Additionally, orthopedic surgery has witnessed substantial decreases in reimbursement, including 23% to 38% in sports medicine procedures,[9] 24% to 43% in orthopedic trauma cases,[10] and 17% to 39% in spine surgery.[11] In the background of all these changes is an amplified pres-sure to increase surgical volume, ensure exceptional patient satisfaction, and, in the setting of academic medicine, conduct groundbreaking research and/or educate the next generation of physicians. Health-care delivery is more complex today than ever before, and orthopedic surgery is certainly no exception.

With increasing competition and a growing demand (and desire) for success—both personally and professionally—in an ever-changing and intricate health-care land-scape, leadership becomes ever more critical. The issues discussed above cannot be addressed adequately without strong leadership. The best leaders adapt with the times, thriving at solving paradoxical demands (do more with less) and disruptive change.[12] However, this requires hard work and practice, not just luck or good fortune. Indeed, the most successful orthopedic surgery leaders know this firsthand. However, what can differentiate the good from great current orthopedic surgery leaders and up-and-coming orthopedic surgery leaders of tomorrow? Coaching.

What Is Coaching?

Coaching "involves inquiry, encouragement, and accountability to increase self-awareness, motivation, and the capacity to take effective action."[13] Indeed, coaching is a core component to any participant in a competitive endeavor seeking to perform at their best, whether it be in athletics, music, or health care (eg, orthopedic surgery). Coaching can be the difference maker that takes something mediocre or "pretty good" to excellent or the "next level"; the value of coaching cannot be understated. As legendary National Football League coach Pete Carroll of the Seattle Seahawks once said, "[e]ach person holds so much power within themselves that needs to be let out. Sometimes they just need a little nudge, a little direction, a little support, a little coaching, and the greatest things can happen."[14] Coaching can be peer-to-peer or through a professional coach.

Peer-to-peer coaching focuses on interactions between individuals who are roughly at the same stage and position in their career but who do not have any oversight or authority over each other. Given the "insider" knowledge similar individuals share in this setting, reflection on current practices within a given organization or industry may be more tangible and of value. "Best" practices can be shared among peers and accountability may be stronger. Some argue the leadership development skills gained in a peer-to-peer setting, especially group settings, are preferable to other forms of one-to-one coaching (eg, professional coaching).[15] It can also be cost-effective.[16]

The International Coaching Federation, the leading global organization for coaches and coaching, defines coaching in the professional setting "as partnering with [individuals] in a thought-provoking and creative process that inspires them to maximize their personal and professional potential."[17] In contrast to peer-to-peer coaching, one-to-one coaching typically involves a professional "outsider" with more motivational and broad-based expertise in optimizing individual personal and professional performance than subject matter expertise. Professional coaches tend not to be directly related to the function of the given company but can help provide direction, improve performance, and guide conversations around opening up opportunities and removing barriers to progress.

How Does Coaching It Fit into Orthopedic Surgery?

Inherently, most orthopedic surgeons are competitive individuals. They pushed themselves throughout undergraduate studies and medical school just for the opportunity to train in the field. Once matched into residency, they pushed themselves even harder, through early mornings and late nights, to learn the "ins and outs" of delivering high value musculoskeletal care in the clinic and the operating room. After graduating residency, many continue educational pursuits by pursuing subspecialty training before embarking on their career as an attending orthopedic surgeon.

Even after completing all necessary clinical training, doubt can creep in. Am I doing this right? Is this the best approach for my patient? What if this procedure goes poorly or the clinical outcome is not what was expected? Pair these concerns with a changing health-care delivery landscape with evolving payment mechanisms and personal responsibilities and all of a sudden, performance can falter, patients may suffer, family and personal life becomes secondary, and burnout looms. These concerns can be addressed. As "elite athletes" in medicine, orthopedic surgeons can greatly benefit from coaching, which in turn can help counteract many of the outside forces that may cause a negative "spiraling" effect.

Understanding how coaching can play a positive role in daily life and clinical practice is vital for orthopedic surgeons. In fact, this is paramount because all orthopedic surgeons are leaders, although it is on different scales. At a minimum, orthopedic surgeons are the leaders in their practices, operating rooms, and among patient care teams. On a larger scale, orthopedic surgeons can lead divisions, departments, practices, or even large national or international professional organizations or institutions. Regardless of the "level of leader", coaching can have a positive, lasting impact on performance and well-being. Specifically, coaching can reduce burnout and improve resiliency while also helping to inspire continuous improvement for and optimize performance of an orthopedic surgeon and their team. In the following sections, we touch on these key focus areas.

The Role of Coaching in Addressing Burnout

Burnout is a serious threat to health care, including for physicians at the front lines of care delivery. This is even more true now than ever before with impending workforce shortages, including a projected shortage of 15,800 to 30,200 physicians in the surgical specialties by 2034, including orthopedic surgery.[18] In fact, addressing health-care professional burnout remains a current priority of the United States Surgeon General.[19] When it comes to orthopedic surgery leaders, coaching can play a critical role in reducing burnout.

Although it should not be, burnout can be viewed as weakness or lack of resiliency. Defining burnout as an illness, or condition, may further worsen the stigma; unfortunately, this was recently done by the World Health Organization.[20] Although coaching has been used for many years in the business world, its role in health care is much newer; however, it undoubtedly can play an important role in helping to tackle burnout in a manner that is less stigmatized.[21]

The initial research demonstrating the improvement in physician well-being in the setting of coaching is very promising. In one qualitative study of physicians who participated in 3 to 8 individual coaching sessions, study participants reported increased resilience.[22] Specifically, physicians noted resiliency improvement in 3 key areas: (1) boundary setting and prioritization, (2) self-compassion and self-care, and (3) self-awareness.[22] Further, although indirect, there was a thought that the downstream effect of improved resilience from the coaching session was improved patient care and a better understanding that devaluing self-care in exchange for increased time spent care of others is a common, but avoidable, cause of burnout.[22]

Another study of 80 surgeons randomized to receive monthly professional coaching for 6 months or not further demonstrated improvement in burnout symptoms and resiliency among those receiving coaching.[23] Interestingly, once these sessions ended, surgeons exhibited a return of their burnout symptoms but continued resiliency improvement,[23] suggesting that ongoing coaching may be important to optimize the benefits of coaching on burnout symptom management. Another similar study of non-surgeons found similar results, including improvement in quality of life as well.[13] Overall, however, further work into the frequency and duration of coaching sessions, as well as other characteristics (eg, does "style" make a difference?), is needed.

The reality is that orthopedic surgeons face constant stressors at home and at work that negatively affect mental well-being and can lead to burnout. Although many pursue medicine, including orthopedic surgery, because of a "calling" to help others and make a positive difference in others' lives, in some cases they do so at the sacrifice of their own well-being. However, burnout can be addressed successfully and better managed. One framework highlights that overcoming burnout requires 4 steps: (1) prioritize your own health, (2) focus on aspects of a situation that can change or be addressed and not those that are fixed (ie, "control the controllable"), (3) reduce involvement in stressful activities and exposure to stressful relationships as much as possible, and (4) seek out and focus on the interpersonal connections that are helpful.[24] Coaching can play an integral role in ensuring that orthopedic surgery leaders successfully navigate these 4 steps in a manner that allows them to thrive in their various roles, leading to improved personal and professional outcomes.

Not Being Satisfied—the Role of Coaching in Improving Performance, Inspiring a Drive to "Be Better," and Making Progress Every Day

The orthopedic surgery leader has a remarkable number of tasks and commitments each day. From clinical work in the operating room or clinic setting to hospital, practice, and division or departmental policy meetings to personal responsibilities, 24 hours in a day may never seem like enough. As noted above, coaching can help alleviate symptoms of burnout that may occur because of this overwhelming schedule. However, coaching can do much more than just help alleviate burnout; coaching can also improve performance and reignite a passion for continuous improvement and success because it relates to patient outcomes.

Unlike teaching, which is more of a one-way knowledge transfer, or mentoring, which offers guidance broadly and is more instructional in nature, coaching in surgery fosters a dialog that leads to the coachee, or surgeon, making the final decision and arriving at solutions himself or herself. From a clinical standpoint, coaching can provide a way for surgeons to reflect on their technical skills in the operating room or clinical outcomes in a nonjudgmental manner, allowing for a more in depth evaluation of what may be going right or wrong. Action can then be taken to correct any underlying issues in a more collaborative way. If professional coaching is used, the coach plays an important role in helping to frame the issues, whereas in peer-to-peer coaching, trust can be further built among surgeons of similar stature because they discuss challenging cases, patient outcomes, or technical "tips and tricks." Ultimately, this can lead to better patient outcomes, although further research is needed in this area given the wide variation in study designs and coaching interventions evaluated to date in the literature.[25]

Although the research on the impact of coaching on performance is limited within health care, there is a growing body of literature more broadly focused on assessing coaching on performance in organizational settings. For example, a recent meta-analysis asking the question "does coaching work?" found that coaching significantly improved individual performance and skills in an organizational context.[26] In addition, 7 out of 10 people in organization and leadership settings reported improved work performance, relationships, and more effective communication skills secondary to coaching.[27] However, what may best demonstrate the value of coaching on performance is a study of 31 managers who underwent standard managerial training followed by one-on-one executive coaching for either weeks.[28] Although training improved productivity by 22.4%, the addition of coaching improved productivity by 88.0%.[28] Given the complex organizations orthopedic surgery leaders find themselves in on a daily basis, we suspect that such findings are transferrable. As such, we believe coaching should be considered a way to drive improved performance globally, whereas the impact of coaching on specific performance indicators in an orthopedic surgery setting require further scholarly inquiry.

Outside of the operating room or clinic setting, coaching can help orthopedic surgery leaders engage with tasks or goals that may seem insurmountable in a much more productive manner. For example, large culture change initiatives, structural reorganization, and/or other high-level decisions that influence individuals and organizations can be overwhelming and falter without a clear and cohesive plan of action. In many cases, coaching can play a pivotal role in helping the orthopedic surgery leader reflect on the issue at hand and then define incremental goals and behavior adjustments to make the much larger initiative a success.

Important to remember is that coaching for the orthopedic surgery leader is not meant to be remedial or evidence of "failure." In contrast, coaching can help highlight elements of excellent performance and help orthopedic surgeon leaders try to mirror the skills used in achieving such outcomes in situations where there is an opportunity for improvement. Indeed, the most successful coaches focus on "best performances" as a means of driving improved performance more broadly.[21] Further, while much is learned during medical training, leadership and performance enhancement skills are typically not a core focus. Thus, despite a desire among many orthopedic surgery leaders to "be the best," many of the nonorthopedic skills needed are lacking; coaching can help fill the void and inspire individuals to make constant adjustments and improve each day to reach their ultimate goals.

Being Coached Versus Being a Coach

Orthopedic surgery leaders are uniquely positioned in that they both can benefit from coaching and also, in many instances, can be a coach as well, especially in peer-to-peer settings.

> **Box 1**
> **Eight practices of highly successful surgeons that coaching can help reinforce or improve on**
>
> Passion for performance improvement
>
> Reciprocity of roles and relationships
>
> Attitude resilience
>
> Communication with mutual understanding
>
> Time/life management using rhythm
>
> Inspiring to shared goals
>
> Complex problem-solving through simplicity
>
> Energy for personal and practice wellness
>
> *From* Smith, Jeffrey M. MD, FACS, CPC. Surgeon Coaching: Why and How. Journal of Pediatric Orthopaedics: July 2020 - Volume 40 - Issue - p S33-S37 https://doi.org/10.1097/BPO. 0000000000001541.

Typically, in order to become an orthopedic surgery leader, one must excel at demonstrating advanced expertise in orthopedic surgery knowledge while also having the technical skills needed to thrive clinically. Further, many orthopedic surgery leaders develop into key opinion leaders based on their scholarly endeavors in conjunction with their clinical acumen. However, as orthopedic surgeons demonstrate their successes in these areas, they often find themselves in positions of leadership without much training or knowledge of how to be an effective leader. Thus, coaching on how to become and remain an effective leader is crucial to consistent success and progress of the respective group or organization. This is especially true because there has been an ongoing shift toward the role of managers becoming that of a coach, leading to more question-asking, support, and career development focus.[29] Therefore, now more than ever, utilizing professional coaching can be vital for orthopedic surgery leaders looking to optimize their team's performance.

At the same time that professional coaching can be beneficial for orthopedic surgery leaders, peer-to-peer coaching can be equally as helpful. Across institutions and practices, many orthopedic surgery leaders may face similar, yet slightly different challenges. Additionally, few individuals have the experience of being an orthopedic surgery leader and navigating the challenges such individuals face. As such, sharing experiences openly and without judgement in the setting of offering guidance and asking open-ended questions can lead to progress across institutions. Further, the benefit of being seen as "equals" can create a sense of camaraderie among a group of peers. Not only is such peer-to-peer coaching cost-effective, it can also be effective in getting tasks or goals accomplished.

Final Thoughts

Being in a position of leadership within orthopedic surgery is a privilege. However, it can also be understandably stressful and overwhelming at times. In today's healthcare landscape, there is a paradoxical demand to "do more with less." Further, there is an expectation that orthopedic surgery leaders are always available, patient outcomes and satisfaction are flawless (or nearly flawless), and that disruptive changes in the system (eg, staffing issues or decreased reimbursements) are ones that you—as the orthopedic surgery leader—should be able to "solve" or at least adapt to in your role. At the same time, personal responsibilities and commitments remain.

These multitude of challenges are real and can lead to burnout, poor performance, and declining mental and physical health. Although it is not a "magic bullet" solution, coaching can be a valuable mechanism to address burnout, inspire individuals to push themselves to "be better" each day, and develop and refine leadership skills. Coaching can reignite a passion among orthopedic surgery leaders to strive for continuous improvement, both for themselves and for those around them.

Although many frameworks exist to understand the positive role coaching can have for orthopedic surgery leaders, one developed by a fellow orthopedic surgeon highlights the 8 key practices individuals can use to optimize their performance, and, in our opinion, the performance of those around them (**Box 1**).[21] Using this framework as a guide, leaders can ensure they are approaching the complexities of their professional and personal lives in a manner that optimizes outcomes. Further, if there are areas that an individual struggles in, he or she now recognizes this and can seek professional coaching expertise or peer-to-peer coaching to address the deficiency.

With the level of expertise, technical skills, and practice needed to excel, orthopedic surgeons can be compared with high-level athletes or musicians. As such, coaching can be considered a key component of pushing boundaries and taking orthopedic surgery leaders to the "next level," which will positively influence not only them but also their colleagues and patients. The positive value of coaching for orthopedic surgery leaders should not be underestimated.

REFERENCES

1. Singhal S, Radha M, Vinjamoori N. The next frontier of care delivery in healthcare. McKinsey & Company; 2022. Available at: https://www.mckinsey.com/industries/healthcare-systems-and-services/our-insights/the-next-frontier-of-care-delivery-in-healthcare. Accessed September 6, 2022.

2. Musculoskeletal health. World Health Organization. 2022. Available at: https://www.who.int/news-room/fact-sheets/detail/musculoskeletal-conditions. Accessed September 7, 2022.

3. Ollove M. Health worker shortage forces states to scramble. The pew charitable trusts. 2022. Available at: https://www.pewtrusts.org/en/research-and-analysis/blogs/stateline/2022/03/25/health-worker-shortage-forces-states-to-scramble. Accessed September 6, 2022.

4. Shanafelt TD, West CP, Sinsky C, et al. Changes in burnout and satisfaction with work-life integration in physicians and the general US working population between 2011 and 2020. Mayo Clin Proc 2022;97(3):491–506.

5. Daniels AH, DePasse JM, Kamal RN. Orthopaedic surgeon burnout: diagnosis, treatment, and prevention. J Am Acad Orthop Surg 2016;24(4):213–9.

6. Williams ES, Rathert C, Buttigieg SC. The personal and professional consequences of physician burnout: a systematic review of the literature. Med Care Res Rev 2020;77(5):371–86.

7. Rathert C, Williams ES, Linhart H. Evidence for the quadruple aim: a systematic review of the literature on physician burnout and patient outcomes. Med Care 2018;56(12):976–84.

8. Robeznieks A. Prior authorization is a major practice burden. How do you compare? American Medical Association (AMA). 2018. Available at: https://www.ama-assn.org/practice-management/prior-authorization/prior-authorization-major-practice-burden-how-do-you. Accessed September 7, 2022.

9. Pollock JR, Richman EH, Estipona BI, et al. Inflation-adjusted medicare reimbursement has decreased for orthopaedic sports medicine procedures: analysis from 2000 to 2020. Orthop J Sports Med 2022;10(2). 23259671211073722.

10. Haglin JM, Lott A, Kugelman DN, et al. Declining medicare reimbursement in orthopaedic trauma surgery: 2000-2020. J Orthop Trauma 2021;35(2):79–85.

11. Haglin JM, Zabat MA, Richter KR, et al. Over 20 years of declining Medicare reimbursement for spine surgeons: a temporal and geographic analysis from 2000 to 2021. J Neurosurg Spine 2022;1–8.

12. Kaiser RBR. The best leaders are versatile ones. Harv Business Rev 2020. Available at: https://hbr.org/2020/03/the-best-leaders-are-versatile-ones. Accessed September 6, 2022.

13. Dyrbye LN, Shanafelt TD, Gill PR, et al. Effect of a professional coaching intervention on the well-being and distress of physicians: a pilot randomized clinical trial. JAMA Intern Med 2019;179(10):1406–14.

14. Jenks J. Seahawks coach Pete Carroll leads players with positive approach. The Seattle Times. 2014. Available at: https://www.seattletimes.com/sports/seahawks/seahawks-coach-pete-carroll-leads-players-with-positive-approach/. Accessed September 8, 2022.

15. Steinberg B, Watkins MD. The Surprising Power of Peer Coaching. Harv Business Rev 2021. Available at: https://hbr.org/2021/04/the-surprising-power-of-peer-coaching. Accessed September 10, 2022.

16. Hauwiller J. Peer coaching can be a win for organizations when everyone plays their part. Forbes. 2021. Available at: https://www.forbes.com/sites/forbescoachescouncil/2021/05/03/peer-coaching-can-be-a-win-for-organizations-when-everyone-plays-their-part/?sh=6b264dca6900. Accessed September 8, 2022.

17. International Coaching Federation (ICF). Empowering the world through coaching. 2022. Available at: https://coachingfederation.org/. Accessed September 9, 2022.

18. Association of American Medical Colleges (AAMC). AAMC report reinforces mounting physician shortage. 2021. Available at: https://www.aamc.org/news-insights/press-releases/aamc-report-reinforces-mounting-physician-shortage. Accessed September 11, 2022.

19. Office of the U.S. Surgeon General. Health Worker Burnout. U.S. Department of Health and Human Services. 2022. Available at: https://www.hhs.gov/surgeongeneral/priorities/health-worker-burnout/index.html.   Accessed September 9, 2022.

20. Berg S. WHO adds burnout to ICD-11. What it means for physicians. American Medical Association (AMA). 2019. Available at: https://www.ama-assn.org/practice-management/physician-health/who-adds-burnout-icd-11-what-it-means-physicians. Accessed September 10, 2022.

21. Smith JM. Surgeon coaching: why and how. J Pediatr Orthop 2020;40(Suppl 1):S33–7.

22. Schneider S, Kingsolver K, Rosdahl J. Physician coaching to enhance well-being: a qualitative analysis of a pilot intervention. Explore (NY) 2014;10(6):372–9.

23. Dyrbye LN, Gill PR, Satele DV, et al. Professional coaching and surgeon well-being. a randomized controlled trial. Ann Surg 2022.

24. Valcour M. Beating burnout. harvard business review. 2016. Available at: https://hbr.org/2016/11/beating-burnout. Accessed September 9, 2022.

25. Skinner SC, Mazza S, Carty MJ, et al. Coaching for surgeons: a scoping review of the quantitative evidence. Ann Surg Open 2022;3(3):e179.

26. Theeboom T, Beersma B, van Vianen AEM. Does coaching work? A meta-analysis on the effects of coaching on individual level outcomes in an organizational context. J Positive Psychol 2014;9(1):1–18.
27. Institute of Coaching. Benefits of Coaching. McLean, Affiliate of Harvard Medical School. 2022. Available at: https://instituteofcoaching.org/coaching-overview/coaching-benefits. Accessed September 18, 2022.
28. Olivero G, Bane KD, Kopelman RE. Executive coaching as a transfer of training tool: effects on productivity in a public agency. Public Pers Manage 1997;26(4):461–9.
29. Ibarra H, Scoular A. The leader as coach. Harv Business Rev 2019;110–9.

Mentorship

Enabling Medical Leaders Through Mentoring

Patrick J. Sweeney, COL, Retired, US Army, PhD[a],*, Joe LeBoeuf, COL, US Army, Retired, PhD[b]

KEYWORDS

- Mentoring • Mentorship • Leader Development • Leadership

KEY POINTS

- Mentoring is important for the development of medical leaders.
- The mentoree is responsible for selecting, establishing, and maintaining mentor releationships.
- Organizations can facilitate mentoring by communicating its importance, encouraging all leaders to engage in mentoring, and providing resources to support mentoring.

INTRODUCTION

Mentorship has proved to be a necessity in all aspects of medicine within the past years.[1]

As this quote suggests, mentoring is an important leader behavior, powerfully relevant in today's volatile, uncertain, complex, and ambiguous world, where virtual and hybrid work conditions have significantly disrupted our social structures, particularly human connection and relational leading, both essential aspects of the medical profession. Developmental programming, characterized by high-quality coaching and mentoring, is an essential activity associated with enabling effective leadership in all forms of organizational life. Mentoring is not just a leader competency but from our perspective, it is foundation to leader development and a significant act of professionalism through organizational stewardship.

Yet, in medical organizations, ".... we have not grown our physicians to be leaders. In fact, we take pride in a system that actually tends to beat out of our doctors any ability they might have as a leader."[2] In effect, medical leaders have neither developed physicians' competencies to lead the necessary precursor for mentorship nor inspired the need for the behavior as a central element of professional, organizational life.

[a] Allegacy Center for Leadership and Character, School of Business, Wake Forest University, P.O. Box 7897, 1834 Wake Forest Road, Winston-Salem, NC 27109, USA; [b] Duke University, Fuqua School of Business, LeadershipMatters LLC, 16535 Flintrock Falls Lane, Charlotte, NC 28278, USA
* Corresponding author.
E-mail address: sweenepj@wfu.edu

Clin Sports Med 42 (2023) 219–231
https://doi.org/10.1016/j.csm.2022.11.006
0278-5919/22/© 2022 Elsevier Inc. All rights reserved.

Mentoring does not seem to receive the attention it should and come to mind for physicians as an intentional behavior, and a lack of this type programming in the medical community is often the rule, and not the exception.

Leading is a behavior that requires attention (eg, mindfulness) to fundamentals and then behaving as a leader with intention to achieve desired individual and collective outcomes. With this as context, this article is organized around several core areas of conversation to bring attention to and make a case for intentional mentoring as a core leader behavior:

- why mentoring is a must (the argument),
- what is mentoring (an operational definition),
- coaching versus mentoring (the differences that matter),
- core principles for effective mentoring (mentoring 101),
- recommendations around building a supportive culture (the ecological "system")

Why Mentoring is a Must: the Argument

Medical professionals need education and training in effective leadership and in the process of leader development. Critical to the leadership role and the leadership development process is the capability to mentor future professionals and leaders in the profession. Mentorship is important in the transmission of the professional identity and mindsets as well as the enhancement of young leaders' knowledge, skills, abilities, and competencies to effectively lead within organizations and the profession. In the mentoring process, both mentors and mentees grow as leaders that result in enhanced individual and organizational performance.[3] "A number of scholars and certainly numerous practitioners have touted the importance of mentorship in promoting leader development."[4] Mentoring enhances leader efficacy and is predictive of leader's performing at higher levels.

Mentoring is not just essential for the development of leadership in the profession but it has important second-order and third-order effects pertaining to significant individual and organizational outcomes. At the individual-level, mentoring positively influences career choices, enhances engagement, increases job satisfaction, bolsters motivation to continue to improve, and enhances well-being. Mentors help individuals learn: to demonstrate care, concern and understanding for others, core in building trust; to cultivate effective relationships to enable others to be their best selves; and inspires continuous personal change, empowering capacity in the ever-changing work context.[5] Similarly, at the organizational-level, mentoring enhances retention and productivity.[6]

What is Mentoring: an Operational Definition

Mentorship is far more than just teaching and coaching. It is about trust, friendship, and in the end — wisdom.[7]

The notion of mentoring has been around for well more than a millennium. Its historical roots come from a character named Mentor (from Greek mythology), an Ithacan noble, and friend of the Greek hero Odysseus, in Homer's epic story *The Odyssey*. Homer asked Mentor to tutor his son, Telemachus, when he went off to the Trojan War, and it is the "deep" personal relationship that developed between these 2 that has served as the foundational basis for the notion of mentorship. "Thus 'mentor' became a verb in the English language with its own meaning: to impart wisdom and share knowledge with a younger colleague."[8] It has emerged as a significant leader behavior, built around the quality of a relationship. Most scholars agree that these relationships are dynamic, learning partnerships, asymmetric, yet reciprocal, with significant benefits to both mentor and protégé (mentee).[9]

At its core, mentoring is primarily good leadership and is the process of building human capital through the creation of effective relationships that enable the transfer of knowledge, experience, and wisdom to others, strengthening leadership capacity and enhancing work (eg, professional) identity. As an act of *generativity*, mentoring passes on a professional legacy, wisdom to the following generations of professionals, and builds a sense of what it means to be a professional. It is a significant demonstration of a stewardship investment in others and the organization, the outcome of responsible leadership in the profession.

With this in mind, mentoring, as good interpersonal leadership is typically defined as "a committed, long-term relationship in which a senior person (mentor – and more experienced) supports the personal and professional development of a junior person (mentee – and less experienced)."[10] In a more expansive definition, the Army describes mentoring as "the proactive development of each subordinate through observing, coaching, teaching, developmental counseling, and evaluating that results in people being treated with fairness and equal opportunity. Mentoring is an inclusive process for everyone under a leader's charge."[11]

Mentoring, in a professional context, is different than just any old voluntary activity. Leading, mentoring, and developing the future leaders of the profession are requirements for membership in a profession, and thus carries a sense of mandate. Therefore, with these considerations in mind, we define mentoring, in the medical professional context, as follows:

> Good leadership, characterized by a "teaching" mindset practiced by senior members to assist in shaping a professional identity and elevating the leadership knowledge, skills, abilities, and competencies of junior members to enhance the profession.

It is a core behavior of professional stewardship, and an essential leadership competency.

Coaching Versus Mentoring: the Differences that Matters

".... the ultimate test for a leader is not whether he or she makes smart decisions and takes decisive action, but whether he or she *teaches* others to be leaders and builds and organization that can sustain its success even when he or she is not around."[12]

The root meaning of doctor is "doceo"—I teach. Kouzes and Posner state the best leaders are the best teachers.[13] Professions ought to be populated by leaders who embrace a "teachable point of view" in all their activities.[14] Coaching and mentoring, at the end of the day, are about teaching and the passing on of "stories." This is the way that leaders pass on our legacies to others, share wisdom that strengthens organizations, the profession, through an investment in others.[15] David Gergen, in his recent book, *Hearts Touched with Fire* states, "It is hard to overstate how much difference a dedicated, first-class coach, mentor, or role model can make in molding the leaders of tomorrow. No matter how many classes in management and leadership young people take, there is no substitute for person-to-person relationships with older people who have learned the arts of navigating through rough seas."[16]

Even with these similarities, there are important differences that required care in clarity on effects desired as one chooses between these 2 important leadership development activities—coaching and mentoring are different behaviors and achieve different outcomes and effects.[17] In the main, the difference between coaching and mentoring can most readily be differentiated through the notion of *transactional* versus *transformational* behavior. Coaching is about one's job, and doing that well, whereas mentoring is about one's career and professional role.

Coaching is fundamentally a transactional process, whose purpose is to "guide learning or improvement skills."[18] Coaching is all about developing competencies and is typically focused on building knowledge, skills, and abilities, or improving performance in a specific area of endeavor, assessed, and directed by the coach. Coaching identifies behaviors that need improvement with the intent to create the conditions for a higher level of performance. Coaching is heavy on telling with feedback, and usually concentrates on short-term needs.

Mentoring, however, subsumes coaching (eg, good mentors understand and practice good coaching skills as prerequisites for an invitation to mentor) but elevates the interaction in a more transformational way with a long-term focus. Mentoring is a deeper relationship—a more experienced person agrees to support the development of a less experienced person (mentoree) beyond just knowledge, skills, and abilities but to "provide guidance focused on professional and personal growth."[18] Mentoring has other broader applications than coaching including education on the organization and culture, identity transformation, and the acceleration of development as a leader.

As Kathy Kram, in her seminal work on mentoring suggests, mentoring is not limited to the development of a small subset of skills that characterizes coaching but it is really focused on the whole person, that includes both career and psychosocial functions essential to individual and organizational effectiveness, and in our case, sustainment of the profession.[19] Mentoring also contributes significantly to other aspects of organizational effectiveness and medical professional life: the inspiration and capacity to *lead* and *develop* others to lead in the profession, and the socialization and development of the unique *professional identity*, which is critically necessary to sustain the profession over time and the building of capacity to meet the increasing demands of professional practice.[20]

From this conversation, we hope it is clear that mentoring matters, as a leader behavior much different than coaching, particularly in the way it develops leader capacity, which influences well-being, and other kinds of positive impacts that enables personal, organizational, and professional capacity across all manner of human flourishing. With this said, there are some very practical, well-researched guidelines for effective mentor and mentoree behavior that will create an important developmental partnership. The basics of being a good mentor and mentee are covered in the next section.

CORE PRINCIPLES FOR EFFECTIVE MENTORING: MENTORING 101
Types of Mentoring

Informal mentoring. Informal mentoring takes place naturally in day-to-day interactions with peers, senior physicians, residents, students, and members of professional associations or clubs. These organic mentoring opportunities are unstructured and do not have specific development objectives. With informal mentoring, the mentee and mentors are free to choose who they want to engage with to promote development.[21] Most mentoring takes place in an informal manner.

Formal mentoring. Formal mentoring takes place intentionally as part of an organization's people development system. The mentoring engagements are structured, have oversight, and are designed to meet specific development objectives. In formal mentoring, the mentee might be assigned a mentor or may have some choice in selecting a mentor.[6]

The Mentoring Process

Selecting a mentor. The first step in selecting a mentor is to enhance your self-awareness regarding your purpose, values, career vision, strengths, and areas needing improvement. This can be done through reflection and seeking feedback from others.[22] These reflective exercises serve as an informal developmental needs assessment. Next, look for potential mentors, both inside and outside of your organization, who possess the expertise and experience to meet your developmental needs, have personality types that you can work with, share similar interests, have good reputations, and possess the desire to assist in developing others. The goal is to build a network of mentors to meet your developmental needs and provide you various perspectives.[23] After identifying potential mentors, approach them to ask if they will consider being your mentor. If person agrees to become your mentor, you now assume responsibility for establishing and maintaining the relationship. If the person turns down, do not be hurt or frustrated because the potential mentor may not have the time or energy to be an effective mentor.[24] Remember, you are responsible for your development and selecting a mentor to serve as a guide enhances your growth as a professional. Outlined below are best practices for effectively managing a mentor relationship.

Proactively schedule meetings—the mentee is responsible for scheduling meetings with mentors. The meeting rhythm should be discussed during the initial meeting and be included in the charter.

Cocreate the relationship charter—during the first couple of meetings, codevelop a relationship charter with the mentor addressing purpose, norms, expectations, goals, vision for success, your goals, and meeting rhythm. The charter provides structure to accelerate the development of the relationship.[25]

Setting the agenda—the mentee creates the agenda for each meeting, based on developmental needs, questions, commitments from previous meeting, or recent experiences.[26] Be sure to send the agenda to the mentor a couple of days in advance so he or she has the time to prepare for the meeting.

Drive the developmental action planning—the mentee is responsible for creating and executing developmental action plans that include goals, subgoals, timelines, and metrics.[27] The mentor assists in guiding action planning and execution.

Meet commitments—the mentee is responsible for the execution of the development plan, doing prework, and fulfilling all commitments to prepare for each session.[28] If the mentee cannot fulfill a commitment, he or she needs to let the mentor know as soon as possible.

Be loyal and grateful—the mentor is providing you gifts of wisdom and time to assist in your development. Mentees need to protect confidentiality, support the mentor, and express appreciation for the mentor's time and knowledge.[29]

Mentoring relationships are invaluable to your developmental as a professional.[30] Work hard to ensure the relationship is mutually beneficial and the mentor's investment in you is yielding results. Remember, build a network of mentors to meet development needs while considering the time you have to effectively manage the relationships.

Becoming a mentor. The first step to becoming a mentor is to determine if you would serve as a good role model, possess the motivation to develop others, have the time to invest in mentoring others, and have the flexibility in your schedule to be available to mentees. If your current situation prevents you from establishing mentoring relationships, capitalize on day-to-day opportunities to informally mentor people. Next, after you determine you possess the qualities, motivation, and time to mentor others, develop or hone your mentoring skills through self-study or with organization resources. Third, based on your experience, expertise, interests, and personality, determine the young professionals who are most likely to benefit from your mentorship. Once you have set the conditions for being a successful mentor, you are ready to start mentoring. Outlined below are best practices in being an effective mentor.[31]

1. Invest time to build trust—take time to share information about yourself and to learn about the mentee. The intent is to get to know each other and start building trust before starting the mentoring partnership.
2. Create a charter—take time during the first couple of sessions to jointly develop a charter, which establishes the framework for the relationship regarding purpose, vision for success, norms, roles, expectations, goals based on mentee's needs, and meeting rhythm. The charter sets the conditions for creating a safe learning environment and accelerating the development of trust within the mentoring partnership. This is why the charter should be completed within the first couple of sessions.
3. Empower the mentee—in assuming control of his or her development, scheduling meetings, setting the agenda, creating, and executing developmental action plans.
4. Be the guide—the mentor's role is to listen, ask reflective questions to guide the mentee in creating developmental plans, sharing insights, providing candid actionable feedback, being available to answer questions, and holding the mentee accountable for executing plans.
5. Be a role model—engage in exemplary leadership, maintain competence, be professional, maintain confidentiality, and be loyal to the organization and mentee.

Being a mentor has many positive outcomes to include a sense of satisfaction in contributing to the future of the profession, enhanced self-awareness and growth, collegiality, and a sense of fulfillment in creating a legacy by developing younger members of the profession.[32] True impact as a professional comes from mentoring others to be motivated, dedicated, and engaged members of the profession.

The typical phases of mentoring. Mentoring relationships evolve through predictable stages as they mature. It is important to note that mentoring relationships evolve over years, there is no set time for stages to emerge, and the stages are likely to overlap to some degree. Moreover, some mentoring relationships may not successfully move out the establishing a relationship phase. This is all right as long as the mentee has multiple mentors. Outline in **Table 1** is a simple evolution of the stages of a typical mentoring relationship with roles and key functions for each stage.[33]

Table 1 Typical stages for a mentoring relationship			
Stage	**Mentee's Role**	**Mentor's Role**	**Key Functions**
Establishing the relationship and beginning the journey	Novice	Guide and coach	• Build trust • Create charter • Set development plan
Flourishing	Protégé	Mentor	• Realize development • Connection to network • Advocate for growth challenges
Maturity	Friend and legacy	Friend and mentor	• Maintain friendship • Mentee becomes mentor to others

Data from Kopser, G. J. Mentoring in the Military: Overview and Recommendations for the Individual. Cambridge, MA: Kennedy School of Government, Harvard University; 2002.

Mentoring Functions

Identity development. Mentors play an important role in assisting a mentee in shaping his or her professional identity.[34] The mentor must role model the standards of the profession to include maintaining unique expertise, upholding the profession's ethical standards and holding others accountable, contributing to the profession's body of knowledge, and being a steward of the profession.[35] By serving as a role model and through discussions on the importance of the profession's expectations regarding maintain competence, ethical practice, contributing to the body of knowledge, and investing in service to ensure the future of the profession, the mentor helps the mentee solidify his or her professional identity.

Career development. Mentors offer mentees guidance and coaching on handling their current roles and also to prepare for future roles. These role and career discussions are important because they assist in shaping, in mentees, the mindsets necessary for a satisfying and successful career. Mentors serve as an important source to assist mentees in outlining their career paths and identifying key positions and experiences necessary to reach their career goals.[27] Moreover, mentors can serve as advocates to help mentees secure key developmental experiences or roles to promote career growth as well as introducing them to their networks. Finally, mentors assist mentees in effectively navigating the organization's systems and political environments.[36]

Psychosocial support. Mentors serve as a wonderful source of psychological and social support. They can provide mentees advice on how to handle tough issues (professional and personal), encouragement to handle challenges, put setbacks into perspective to promote learning, provide nonjudgmental feedback, and bolster confidence through positive regard.[36]

Mentoring derailers

Both the mentor and mentee need vigilance in identifying and countering potential derailers to their relationship. These derailers, if left unchecked, have the potential to significantly reduce the effectiveness of the mentoring relationship and possibly destroy the relationship. Outlined below are common derailers to mentoring relationships.

Mentee derailers. Mentees need to ensure they are ready to enter a mentoring relationship by assuming ownership and cultivating an openness to being guided by a mentor. Outlined below are mentee' behaviors or mindsets that could adversely affect the mentoring relationship:[31]

1. Failure to take ownership of your development—this can lead to overreliance on the mentor or a nonfocused development plan, which yields minimal developmental results.

   Counter: Assume responsibility for your development by setting your goals and creating plans to achieve them. View the mentor as a guide and not the driver.

2. Expecting the mentor to solve your problems—the mentor is a guide to assist you in creating solutions to your problems and creating developmental plans to reach your goals.

   Counter: When dealing with a problem, remember it is your responsibility to solve it and that the mentor is one source of support to do this.

3. Lack of openness—a mentee's openness to the mentor's perspectives and suggestions is critical for learning and the relationship to flourish. If the mentee

demonstrates a lack of receptivity to the mentor's suggestions or guidance, he or she is likely to feel the relationship is a waste of valuable time and end it.

Counter: When the mentor is sharing suggestions or offering guidance, use reflective listening to ensure you fully understand the suggestions or guidance. Moreover, remember the mentor has wisdom and your best interests at heart when providing you with guidance or suggestions.

4. Lack of transparency—candid and transparent communication is critical for building trust, exploring developmental needs, and completing developmental plans. Failure to share your true needs, goals, feelings, or status in meeting commitments hinders the development of trust and decrements the effectiveness of mentoring.

Counter: If you find yourself holding back your feelings, true reactions, or information from the mentor, ask yourself why you are doing it. If you determine the reasons to be out of avoiding embarrassment or a threat to your ego, remind yourself the mentor cares about you, has been in your position, and wants you to develop into an effective professional.

5. Breaking confidentiality—sharing the mentor's experiences, true feelings, and thoughts with others breaks confidentiality of the relationship and destroys trust. For a mentoring relationship to work, it must be a safe place where both the mentee and mentor can share experiences and candid thoughts.

Counter: Be sure confidentiality is address in the charter and remind yourself what is said in the mentoring relationship, stays in the mentoring relationship. If people ask you about the mentoring relationship, talk generalities regarding the benefits and never specifics that are discussed.

Mentor derailers. Mentors play a key role in creating a safe, nonjudgmental, and trusting environment conducive to development. Below are some derailers that adversely affect the mentoring relationship mentors need to watch for.[37]

1. Failing to earn mentee's trust—without the mentee's trust, he or she will not allow you to influence or guide his or her development. Trust is earned over time and takes both parties willing to be vulnerable to each other.

Counter: Invest time at the beginning of the relationship to start building trust, complete the charter, and conduct periodic check-ins on the relationship to see what each party can do to enhance trust.

2. Failing to create a safe environment—if the mentee does not feel psychologically safe in the mentoring relationship, he or she will likely engage in guarded communication, withhold information, and have a defensive approach to achieving developmental goals, which inhibits the development.

Counter: Mentors should think before they give feedback to ensure it is nonjudgmental and targeting an idea or plan and not the mentee. Moreover, be sure the norms created in the charter create a psychologically safe climate.

3. Assuming ownership of the mentee's journey—if the mentor starts to direct the mentee's developmental journey, the mentee is likely to become dependent or withdrawal from the relationship.[38]

Counter: Before a session, remind yourself that your role is as a guide. During the session, use questions to get the mentee to think deeper or to guide toward a solution.

After the session, conduct an after-action review to determine if you were directing mentee actions or guiding them. Remember, the mentee's discovery learning is a key component of development.

4. Failure to hold mentee accountable—if the mentor does not hold the mentee accountable for meeting commitments and completing action plans, then the development is greatly hindered.

Counter: Engage in developmental accountability to ensure the mentee keeps on track and meets commitments. If the mentee fails to meet commitments, explore the process used and refine it. The focus is on development and learning and not punishing the mentee. Moreover, remind the mentee, if he or she continues in the failure to meet commitment, the relationship will end.

5. *Being unavailable*—if mentee cannot get on the mentor's schedule, then it is hard to move the developmental relationships forward, which creates frustration for the mentee and damages the relationship.

Counter: Block and protect time on your schedule for your mentoring sessions. If outside sources are adding uncertainty to your schedule, be creative in using mealtimes and virtual sessions to complete the sessions.

Engaging in best practices for managing effective mentor relationships and being aware of potential derailers, can assist both mentees and mentors in building effective developmental relationships.

Necessary Organizational Support: The Work Ecology that Matters Shaping a mentoring culture. Mentors, especially leaders, must value the development of people and think that investing in mentoring others enhances the organization and the profession. This underlying belief that mentoring increases the effectiveness of individuals, the organization, and the profession influences leader behavior, how the organization operates, and how it is brought onto the team. Outlined below are some key leader behaviors and organization's practices and systems that will shape a mentoring culture.

1. Leaders pay attention to and engage in mentoring—leaders, especially senior, who focus on and engage in mentoring are sending a strong message to members of the organization that mentoring is important. Moreover, if leaders track mentoring participation and pay attention to mentoring effectiveness metrics, then members realize mentoring is important and are most likely to engage in mentoring themselves.[21]

2. Mentoring is one part of the people development system—establishing mentoring as an important part of the organization's people development system sets the requirement for all to seek out and engage in mentoring of others. People who are not in a formal leadership position can mentor their peers and less experienced members. Furthermore, having mentoring as a key component of the people development system creates an organizational obligation to train all members on how to be a mentor and/or mentee.[39]

3. Mentoring is part of the performance management and promotion systems—making mentoring a performance management objective signal to people that mentoring is important, and it also increases the likelihood of mentoring behavior throughout the organization. Similarly, making mentoring a promotion criterion serves to increase mentoring behavior within the organization while reinforcing the importance of mentoring. Finally, promoting people who value mentoring further bolsters and ensures the continuity of the mentoring culture within the organization.

4. Leaders recognize and reward effective mentors and communicate about its importance—recognition and rewards are powerful reinforcers to shape mentoring behavior within the organization. Leaders need to ensure they are communicating how the mentoring behavior is benefiting people, the organization, and profession to persuade people's beliefs about mentoring. Once people think that mentoring is part of being professional and beneficial, mentoring behavior becomes a habit.

5. Mentoring is part of job announcements and selection criteria—leaders ensure all job announcements have a requirement regarding mentoring. During interviews, the committee asks the candidate to share his or her views on mentoring and how they have mentored others in the past. Selecting people who believe in the value and have engaged in mentoring reinforces the culture of mentoring.

6. Leaders allocate the time and resources—leaders need to ensure there are resources available to conduct mentoring training, people to oversee a formal mentor program if the organization has implemented one, and, most importantly, allocate time for people to engage in training and mentoring.[40]

Informal, formal, or hybrid mentoring program. There are many factors (eg, operational tempo, size of the organization, resources, training-level, people's attitudes) that come into play when determining the type of mentoring program to implement or reinforce within an organization. Leaders should first assess their organization's current mentoring program to determine its effectiveness in contributing to the development of people. Leaders can use the assessment results to improve the current mentoring program and create plans to enhance it. The key is to have some type of mentoring program to develop the organization's most important asset—its people. Outline below are some considerations for each type of program.

1. Informal program—occurring, at some level, in all organizations, minimal cost to implement, and does not require formal oversight. Organizations have the requirement to provide training and assess the number of people participating and the effectiveness. Because there are no set developmental objectives, the assessment challenges increase, and leaders do not have control on what gets developed. Moreover, leaders have the responsibility to ensure the people who need the mentoring the most are engaging with mentors.

2. Formal program—require administrative and technical support, which increases cost. The formal structure allows leaders to establish developmental goals for all mentees, thus ensuring a baseline of development while making assessment easier. A crucial decision is whether to make the program voluntary or mandatory for both mentors and mentees. Research suggest mandatory participation by mentors is not the optimal course of action.[21] Other important considerations for executing a formal mentor program are getting representative feedback for shaping the program, providing training, pairing mentors and mentees, establishing common developmental objectives, by level, and creating the assessment plan.[41]

3. *Hybrid program*—this type of program provides an organization with the flexibility of an informal program combined with the developmental focus of a formal program. Leaders have the ability to scale up or scale back the formal mentoring while still leveraging the benefit of the informal mentoring. Furthermore, leaders could provide mentors engaged in informal mentoring relationships with a small group of key developmental objectives to consider discussing.

Establishing a mentoring culture sets the conditions for effective mentoring within an organization. Each organization has to determine the type of mentoring program (informal, formal, or hybrid) that best fits its developmental and mission needs. Furthermore, providing all members training on being an effective mentee and mentor increases the likelihood of success. Leaders need to continuously communicate about the benefits of the mentoring program and emphasize professionals have an obligation to contribute to the development of the future.

SUMMARY

The mentor sees in the prospective protégé a youthful energy and enthusiasm – we are tempted to call it wide-eyed enthusiasm, to bolster the point – that triggers some primal desire to nurture, to teach and protect.[42]

Bennis and Thomas, in their book, *Geeks and Geezers*, studied outstanding leadership across generations, and developed the notion that one of the key attributes of young and old leaders is called neoteny, defined as the "retention of youthful characteristics in adulthood."[43] Neoteny is maintained by a relationship characterized by a form of bonding, we often call mentoring. If done right, and with care, concern, understanding, respect and fairness, mentoring can be a "life-altering relationship that inspires mutual growth, learning, and development."[44]

Mentoring is important to the development and enhancement of the medical profession and to organizational performance. The challenge is to implement a mentoring program within your organization. Leaders can use this article to assist in training both mentors and mentees. Remind people that the mindsets and skills necessary to become good mentor and mentee improve with practice, thus engage, learn, and improve. The time invested in mentoring relationships enhance patient care, create positive work climates within organizations, improves individual and organizational performance, and creates a brighter future for the medical profession. "Its effects can be remarkable, profound, and enduring, mentoring relationships have the capacity to transform individuals, groups, organizations and communities."[45] Just do it!

DISCLOSURE

The authors have nothing to disclose.

REFERENCES

1. Asuka ES, Halari C, Halari MM. Mentoring in Medicine. A Retrospective Study. Am Scientific Res J Eng Technology Sci (Asrjets) 2016;19(1):43.
2. Hertling M. Growing physician leaders: empowering doctors to improve our Healthcare. Florida Hospital Publications; 2016. p. 7.
3. Desselle SP, Chang H, Fleming G, et al. Design fundamental of mentoring programs for pharmacy professionals (Part 1): Considerations for organizations. Res Social Administrative Pharm 2021;17:441–8.
4. Lester PR, Hannah ST, Harms PD, et al. Mentoring Impact on Leader Development: A Field Experiment. Acad Management Learn Education 2011;10(3):409.
5. Shanafelt T, Trockel M, Rodriquez A, et al. Wellness-Centered Leadership: Equipping Health Care Leaders to Cultivate Physician Well-Being and Professional Fulfillment. Acad Med 2021;96:641–51.
6. Kashiwagi DT, Varkey P, Cook DA. Mentoring programs for Physicians in Academic Medicine: A systematic review. Acad Med 2013;88(7):1029–37.

7. Kopser J. Mentorship in the military – not everybody gets it. Cambridge, MA: Kennedy School of Government; 2002. p. 2.

8. Homer. The Odyssey. trans. Viking: Robert Fagles; 1996. p. 67.

9. Kimball RA. Mentoring for a professional identity. In: Finney NK, Mayfield TO, editors. Redefining the modern military. Naval Institute Press; 2018. p. 146.

10. Center for Creative Leadership. The Handbook of leadership and development. 2nd edition. Jossey-Bass; 2004. p. 92.

11. Department of the Army. US Army, field manual 22-100, Army leadership. Department of the Army; 1999. p. 5–16.

12. Army US. Field manual Army leadership 22-10. Department of the Army; 1999. p. 3.

13. Kouzes J, Posner B. A leader's legacy. Jossey-Bass; 2006.

14. Kouzes J, Posner B. A leader's legacy. Jossey-Bass; 2006. p. 41.

15. Tichy NM, Cohen E. The leadership engine: how winning companies build leaders at every level. Harper Business; 1997.

16. Gergen D. Hearts touched with Fire: how great leaders are made. Simon & Schuster; 2022. p. 46.

17. Thomas N, Saslow S. Improving productivity through coaching and mentoring, learning solutions. Chief Learning Officer; 2007. www.clomedia.com.

18. Kouzes J, Posner B. A leader's legacy. Jossey-Bass; 2006. p. 5.

19. Kram KE. Mentoring at work: developmental relationships in organizational life. New York University Press; 1988.

20. Browne-Ferrigno T, Muth R. Leadership mentoring in clinical practice: Role of socialization, professional development, and capacity building. Educ Administrative Q 2004;40(4):468–94.

21. Desselle SP, Chang H, Fleming G, et al. Design fundamentals of mentoring programs for pharmacy professionals (Part 1): Considerations for organizations. Res Social Adm Pharm 2021;17(2):441–8.

22. Kopser, 2002: 19-21. Mentorship in the Military [Thesis].

23. Ensher E, Murphy S. Power Mentoring: how successful mentors and proteges get the most of their relationships. Jossey-Bass; 2005.

24. Cheng T, Hackworth JM. The "Cs" of mentoring: using adult learning theory and the right mentors to position early-career investigators for success, notes from the association of medical school pediatric department chairs. J Pediatr 2021; 238:6–8.

25. Johnson WB, Ridley CR. The elements of mentoring. 3rd edition. St. Martin's Press; 2018. p. 105–34.

26. Kopser, 2002: 24-32. Mentorship in the Military [Thesis].

27. Cheng TL, Hackworth JM. The "Cs" of Mentoring: Using Adult Learning Theory and the Right Mentors to Position Early-Career Investigators for Success. J Pediatr 2021;238. 6–8.e2.

28. Harvard Business School. Being an effective mentor and a receptive protégé. In: Harvard business essentials: coaching and mentoring. Boston: Harvard Business School Press; 2004. p. 99–112.

29. Kopser, 2002: 34-35. Mentorship in the Military [Thesis].

30. Underhill CM. The effectiveness of mentoring programs in corporate settings: A meta-analytical review of the literature. J Vocational Behav 2006;68:292–307.

31. Harv Business Sch 2004;99–112.

32. Ehrich LC, Hansford B, Tennent L. Formal mentoring programs in education and other professions: A review of the literature. Education Adm Q 2004;40(4): 518–40.

33. Kopser 2002;23–4.
34. Frei E, Stamm M, Buddeberg-Fischer B. Mentoring programs for medical students – a review of the PubMed literature 2000-2008. BMC Med Education 2010;10(32):1–14.
35. Snider DM, Watkins GL. The future of the Army profession. McGraw-Hill Primis Custom Publishing; 2002.
36. Johnson WB, Ridley CR. The Elements of Mentoring. Palgrave Macmillan 2018;1–67.
37. Johnson WB, Ridley CR. The Elements of Mentoring. Palgrave Macmillan 2018;71–101.
38. Sng JH, Pei Y, Tah YP, et al. Mentoring relationships between senior physicians and junior doctors and/or medical students: A thematic review. Med Teach 2017;39(8):866–75.
39. Department of the Army. Leader development FM 6-22. Washington, D.C.: Department of the Army; 2015.
40. Hansford BC, Ehrich LC, Tennent L. Formal Mentoring Programs in Education and other Professions: A Review of the Literature. Educ Adm Q 2004;40(4):518–40.
41. Kashiwagi DT, Varkey P. Mentoring Programs for Physicians in Academic Medicine: A Systematic Review. Acad Med 2013;88(7):1029–37.
42. Bennis W, Thomas R. Geeks and Geezers. Harvard Business School Press; 2002. p. 15.
43. Bennis WG, Thomas RJ, Geeks Geezers. Harvard Business 2002.
44. Ragins BR, Kram KE. The Handbook of mentoring at work: theory, Research and practice. Sage Publications; 2007. chap 1:3.
45. Ragins BR, Kram K. The Handbook of Mentoring at Work: Theory, Research, and Practice.

How to Become a Mentor and Be Good at It

Robin West, MD

KEYWORDS

• Mentoring • Mentorship • Mentor • Mentee • Leadership • Role model

KEY POINTS

• Mentorship can influence and help to shape careers of the next generation of health-care providers.
• Mentors can enhance their personal leadership skills, improve self-awareness, and increase professional credibility through mentorship relationships.
• To be an affective mentor, one must have a growth mindset, be an active listener, promote trust, and set goals.

WHAT IS MENTORING?

Mentoring is a reciprocal, collaborative, and voluntary relationship in which a more experienced person helps to guide the less experienced person with the purpose of development, learning, and career development. A mentor serves as a teacher, counselor, and advocate to a mentee. Mentoring can result in a mutually beneficial professional relationship over time. The intent of mentoring is not usually to rectify weak performance but to help shape a career or to support an individual that shows promise.

TYPES OF MENTORING MODELS

There are a variety of mentoring models. The one-to-one model is the most traditional of all the types of mentoring. Only the mentor and mentee are involved in this type of mentoring, and it is usually a more-experienced individual paired with a less-experienced or younger mentee.

Group mentoring is when one or several mentors work with a group of mentees. Schools and youth programs often apply this model because there is often not enough time or resources to have one mentor for each participant.

Inova MSK Service Line, Washington Nationals, Georgetown University Medical Center, Uniformed Services University of Health Sciences, UVA School of Medicine, Inova Campus, 8100 Innovation Park Drive Suite 110, Fairfax, VA 22031, USA
E-mail address: robin.west@inova.org

Clin Sports Med 42 (2023) 233–239
https://doi.org/10.1016/j.csm.2022.12.003
0278-5919/23/© 2022 Elsevier Inc. All rights reserved.

sportsmed.theclinics.com

Peer mentoring is when participants from either the same role or department or those that have shared or similar experiences, pair up to offer support for each other. This can be a group or a one-on-one mentoring relationship.

Virtual mentoring has become increasingly popular and occurs when the mentorship relationship is established virtually instead of in-person. Using online software, telephone, or email, participants in this type of mentoring can connect virtually without losing the personal touch.

The reverse mentoring relationship is flipped from the traditional model and occurs when the junior employee mentors a more senior professional. This relationship is usually for the younger or junior professional to teach the skills of a new application or technology to the more senior person.

Finally, speed mentoring is a play on speed dating and usually occurs as part of a corporate event or conference. The mentee has a series of one-on-one conversations with a set of different mentors and usually moves from one mentor to the next after a brief meeting. The mentee should come well prepared with questions for advice from the senior level professionals.

WHY BECOME A MENTOR?

Mentoring can enhance your leadership skills and is a chance to pay it forward. It encourages continuous learning and gives you an opportunity to widen your perspective and learn new things. You get a chance to share your experiences for the betterment of others and for your profession. Mentoring can help to improve self-awareness and increase professional credibility. It allows the mentor to build soft skills and boosts coaching and leadership skills. It is an opportunity to shape tomorrow's leaders and to sharpen your personal knowledge. Mentoring can make you challenge your old beliefs and behaviors and can help you to find purpose and passion through strong personal relationships.

WHO YOU SHOULD MENTOR?

Most people can benefit from having or from being a mentor. You should consider mentoring someone who asks for help or is less experienced within your network, a quiet achiever or a natural born leader but may need some guidance, or someone facing a challenge.[1] You should take an active role in identifying mentees.

When someone seeks out a mentor, you should capitalize on their initiative and discuss how consistent mentoring may help them. A promising protégé may be a younger, less-experienced physician in your practice, your hospital system, or in your specialty. The quiet achiever is often the ideal person to mentor. They may be overshadowed by their more assertive colleagues. Keep an eye out for the "unsung" but productive and talented person who may be able to advance in positions of leadership and influence with some guidance. Born leaders who are collaborative, competent, and productive may benefit from mentorship despite already being on a successful career path. Your guidance may help them to reach their pinnacle. People who are either underrepresented minorities or are facing a challenge can often benefit the most from a mentor as the relationship can show possibilities, help to clarify vision, and open doors of opportunity.

CORE SKILLS OF MENTORING

Dr Phillips-Jones has identified 4 core skills that are required for establishing a successful mentorship relationship.[2,3]

Active Listening

Active listening is the most basic mentoring skill. By listening well, you demonstrate to your mentees that their concerns have been heard and understood. As a result, their trust in the relationship will build quickly. There are several observable behaviors that indicate a good listener: encouraging responses, maintaining direct eye contact, nodding your head, leaning in, avoid interrupting, asking appropriate questions, and summarizing the key elements of what was discussed.

Building Trust

The more trust you build, the more committed the mentee will be and the more effective you will be. To become trustable, you must protect their confidences, spend time with them, follow through on your promises, respect their boundaries, admit error, and take responsibility for correcting any mistakes.

Be Encouraging

According to research done by Dr Linda Phillips-Jones, the most valued mentoring skill is giving encouragement. Mentors and mentees at several Fortune 500 companies revealed in interviews that positive verbal reinforcement—praise—was rare and even publicly discounted in their organizations. However, most people admitted that they enjoyed being recognized and receiving positive feedback for accomplishments and abilities as long as the attention was sincere and not overplayed. The interviewees indicated that they wished positive enforcement was a greater part of their organizational cultures.

There are many ways to encourage your mentee. You can point out positive traits, such as perseverance and integrity, in addition to their excellent performance and accomplishments. You can praise them privately or commend them in front of other people. You can write encouraging emails, letters or leave complimentary voice mails. You can express thanks and appreciation.

Identify Barriers and Goals

You should work with your mentee to establish a vision, identify specific goals, and develop a good understanding of the current situation. You should be open and honest regarding your personal and their personal strengths and limitations.

CRITICAL SKILLS OF MENTORING

Dr Phillips-Jones has identified 5 critical skills that are required for establishing a successful mentorship relationship.[2,3]

Educate and Teach New Skills

A key part of mentoring is educating. You can teach your mentee about the "soft" and the "hard" aspects of medicine. The scientific side of medicine is clearly important, and most students will have spent the majority of their time in college, medical school, and residency learning this "hard" side of medicine. The "soft" side may come naturally for some people and may be more difficult for others.

Soft skills are often what separate a good physician from a great one. Soft skills are subjective, intangible, personality-driven, behavioral, and trans-situational, whereas hard skills are rule-based, tangible, objective, and teachable. Soft skills go beyond patient care and involve the ability to work collaboratively with colleagues and incorporate attitude and social acumen. They are harder to teach but a mentor can help to educate their mentee through discussion and demonstration.

Another piece of the education is teaching the mentoring process. The process should be planned initially with specific steps and reviewed with the mentee. Throughout the mentorship, the process should be addressed by verbalizing and documenting each component so that the mentee has a clear understanding of the goals of each step.

Be Inspiring

One thing that separates good mentors from exceptional ones is the ability to inspire their mentees to greatness. You can stimulate your mentees through your own inspiring actions, by helping them identify and observe other inspiring people, and by challenging them to step outside of their comfort zone. You should help your mentee identify their inspiring vision and challenge them to pursue their own form of significance, not necessarily yours. As Vince Lombardi said, "Perfection is not attainable, but if we chase perfection, we can achieve excellence."

Provide Constructive Feedback

In addition to giving frequent and sincere feedback, effective mentors should be willing and able to give mentees corrective feedback. One of the first things you can discuss with your mentees is how they would prefer to receive this feedback. Some people want very direct advice and others want a more indirect form of input. Some mentees want a lot of support and others may be more independent.

When giving feedback, it should be done in private. The feedback should be honest with positive undertones to encourage necessary change. Feedback should be given immediately and should be focused on specific behaviors to be most effective.

Manage Risks

A distinguishing characteristic of effective mentors is their willingness and ability to protect their mentees from disasters. The mentor should attempt to prevent the mentee from making unnecessary mistakes as they learn to take appropriate risks. However, they should encourage their mentee to take thoughtful chances. They should help their mentee recognize the risks in their actions, make suggestions to help them avoid major mistakes in judgement or action, and also be an advocate for them in difficult situations.

Open Doors

Mentors are often in a position to provide visibility to their mentees. By opening doors, you help to put your mentee in the right place at the right time. You can give your mentee an opportunity to meet the right people, show off their skills and expose them to other potential mentors. You can nominate them for certain positions and speak positively about them in front of your colleagues. Since your reputation can be affected by opening these doors of opportunity, you should make sure that your mentee is prepared and is capable and trustworthy. Explain this process to your mentees as part of the development effort.

TEN STEPS TO SUCCESSFUL MENTORING

We have established the benefits of mentoring, who would make a good mentee, and the core and critical skills of mentoring. Dr Wendy Axelrod has developed the 10 steps of successful mentoring.[4]

Step #1: Prepare for Your Role

Recognize your role as a mentor. Understand your motivation to be a mentor, and participate in a mentorship program or create your own.

Step #2: Establish the Relationship

Spend time getting to know your mentee. What are their interests, goals, strengths, and weaknesses? As you start to develop the relationship, focus on finding common ground, identifying your roles and expectation, and set the tone for ongoing work.

Step #3: Set the Direction

What is the objective of the mentorship relationship? Is it career advancement, personal advice, medical and surgical teaching? Goals should be set early. Too many mentorship relationships are derailed when specific and useful goals are not established.

Step #4: Leverage Experience for Development

Experience is a great teacher when it is properly shaped. Share your negative and positive experiences with your mentee. Share your successes and failures. How can you help to develop your mentee? Decide if you need to be hands-on, working with them to develop their mission or targets. Alternatively, can they independently set the goals and seek your advice as needed. You will need to monitor their progress to make sure the mentoring relationship is successful.

Step #5: Expand Growth Using Everyday Psychology

Helping to create lasting growth will rely on the personal makeup of your mentee. By encouraging your mentee to focus on self-reflection and by creating a safe environment for communication will help to cultivate your mentee. You should help your mentee to develop a growth mindset instead of a fixed mindset. People with a growth mindset like challenges, consider failures as an opportunity to grow, find that feedback is usually constructive, and think that attitude and effort determine their abilities. People with a fixed mindset do not like challenges, think that their potential is predetermined, and usually feel most comfortable in status quo environments.

Step #6: Elevate the Power of Questions

You can help to develop your mentee by asking questions that are thoughtful, developmental, and engaging. You should learn how to ask challenging questions with respect and compassion.

Step #7: Diversify the Development Methods

Help your mentee develop well-rounded skills. Offer some unconventional ways for your mentee to grow personally and professionally. Engage in specific training focused on communication skills, practice management, and leadership in and out of the office. Everyone learns in different ways. You will need to understand the right fit for your mentee, tap into a variety of developmental options, and diversify your own growth during this process.

Step #8: Promote Influence Skills

Use your own personal influence skills but also help your mentee to understand and develop their own skills. Influence skills are the key to being a successful leader. These skills are broad based and include active listening, assertiveness, awareness, empathy, critical thinking, intuition, endurance, innovation, negotiation, persuasion, and time management. Help your mentee recognize and learn to use the 4 crucial influence skills: telling, selling, collaborating, and consulting.

Step #9: Address Mentor Challenges

Mentor challenges should be addressed early and throughout the relationship and may include lack of time or commitment, mismatched expectations of the mentee/mentor, outside influencers, geographic separation, or limited or too much structure.

Step #10: Consolidate Learning and Bring Closure

The closing of the mentorship relationship is as important as the opening. It offers the opportunity for growth and reflection of the mentee and the mentor. It is a chance to celebrate the learnings and achievements of the mentees, thank the mentors for their commitment, share lessons learned, and discuss next steps.

CHARACTERISTICS OF A SUCCESSFUL MENTORING RELATIONSHIP

To explore the characteristics of effective mentors and understanding the factors influencing successful and failed mentoring relationships, Dr Straus and her team performed a qualitative study through the Departments of Medicine at the University of Toronto and the University of California, San Francisco, School of Medicine. They conducted individual, semistructured interviews with faculty members from different career streams and ranks and analyzed transcripts of the interviews. The identified 5 key features of a successful mentoring relationship: reciprocity, mutual respect, clear expectations, personal connection, and shared values.[5]

THE DOS OF A SUCCESSFUL MENTOR (BORG)

Throughout her decorated career as a computer scientist, Dr Anita Borg helped to develop the "Dos" of a successful mentor.[1]

Do: Agree on goals and timelines for the mentoring relationship from the outset and put them in writing. Frequently go back to your goals to measure progress, and do not lose sight of the goals.

Do: Act as a colleague first and as an expert second. A know-it-all approach to mentoring can be intimidating and may limit your successes. Keep an open and warm tone so your mentee will feel comfortable asking difficult questions. Listen as much as you speak so their questions and aspirations are always the central focus.

Do: Set realistic expectations. You can provide your protégé advice, opportunities, and access to resources and people but make it clear that it is their dedication, ambition, and integrity that will make them successful.

Do: Expect high performance from the mentee and accelerate his/her learning. Research suggests that the most beneficial mentoring relationships are based on mutual learning, active engagement, and striving to push the leadership capabilities of the mentee.

Do: Listen wholeheartedly! Hear the questions and concerns of your protégé before offering advice and guidance. Establish trust and openness in communication from the start.

Do: Strive to protect the mentee from what you see as major professional errors or missteps but also leave room for him/her to learn from their own experience and mistakes. Make sure that the mentee is not overly dependent on your advice.

Do: Recognize that the mentees' goals are their own and that they may have career goals that differ from the path you chose. Your role as a mentor is to guide; it is up to the mentee to decide what to implement in their career.

Do: Keep an open mind. Cross-gender and cross-cultural mentoring relationships can be very enriching and successful but they require open dialog about the ways gender and culture influence your mentoring relationship and the mentee's role and development in their own personal career path. Educate yourself about the additional barriers to advancement that minorities may face during their life and career.

Do: Educate others about the importance of mentorship. Consider instituting a "reverse mentoring" program where older leaders are educated about specific issues faced by younger staff, and in diversity issues such as race and gender.

Do: Teach your mentee how to become a mentor herself—by example and by encouragement.

DISCLOSURE

I have no commercial or financial conflicts of interest concerning this article.

REFERENCES

1. Borg A., NWITE Mentoring-in-a-Box: Technical Women at Work. Mentoring Basics-A Mentor's Guide to Success, Available at: https://www.bc.edu/content/dam/files/centers/cwf/individuals/pdf/MentorGuide.pdf, 2007. Accessed July 18, 2007.
2. Phillips-Jones L. The New Mentors and Proteges: How to Succeed with the New Mentoring Partnerships. Valley, CA: Grass; 2001.
3. Phillips-Jones L. The Mentor's Guide: How to Be the Kind of Mentor You Once Had—Or Wish You'd Had. CCC/The Mentoring. Valley, CA: Group, Grass; 2003.
4. Axelrod W. 10 steps to successful mentoring. Alexandria (VA): ATD Press; 2019.
5. Straus SE, Johnson MO, Marquez C, et al. Characteristics of successful and failed mentoring relationships: a qualitative study across two academic health centers. Acad Med 2013;88(1):82–9.

How to Be a Mentee
Getting the Most of Your Mentorship

Lance E. LeClere, MD[a], Meghan E. Bishop, MD[b],*

KEYWORDS

• Mentee • Mentor • Protégé • Student

KEY POINTS

• The mentee is the protégé or the trainee engaged in a relationship with the person with expertise, or the mentor.
• The mentee should approach the mentoring relationship willing to listen, learn, discern, and implement.
• It is advantageous for a mentee to have more than one mentor for different aspects and stages of their career and life.
• The mentor-mentee relationship should be a collaborative and rewarding for both parties.

INTRODUCTION

Mentorship is a key part of the development of knowledge and skills in orthopedics. The differences in phases of learning among the classroom, clinical rotations, and actual practice are vast. Mentorship at each of these different phases is important to preparing and enabling a competent, knowledgeable, and well-rounded surgeon. Although the mentor is generally the one in a senior position, experienced in their field, the mentee is the protégé or the trainee engaged in a relationship with the person with expertise. It is often the perception that much of the onus falls on the mentor to impart their wisdom and guidance for successful mentor–mentee relationship; however, the mentee plays a key role. There should be mutual responsibility on both sides to develop a collaborative relationship in order to optimize value in the relationship for both parties.

Mentorship

The importance of mentorship in orthopedics is well recognized. A recent survey of orthopedic residents found that 100% of residents surveyed reported that having a mentor during residency was either critical (63.7%) or advantageous (37.3%).[1] Of

[a] Vanderbilt University Medical Center, 1215 21st Avenue South, MCE South Tower Suite 4200, Nashville, TN 37232, USA; [b] Rothman Orthopaedic Institute, 645 Madison Avenue, 3rd and 4th Floors, New York, NY 10022, USA
* Corresponding author.
E-mail address: meghanbishop2@gmail.com

Clin Sports Med 42 (2023) 241–248
https://doi.org/10.1016/j.csm.2022.12.004
0278-5919/23/© 2023 Elsevier Inc. All rights reserved.
sportsmed.theclinics.com

Table 1
Criteria-based decision-making steps for identifying a mentor[6]

Step 1. Identify your goal	Consider why you want a mentor Define what you hope to achieve as your end result
Step 2. Create a list of criteria	Identify the qualities you want in a mentor
Step 3. Determine what qualities are "must haves" (Musts)	Select those requirements that are nonnegotiable from your list
Step 4. Rank the remaining criteria (Wants)	Rank order the remaining criteria in order of importance to you
Step 5. List possible options	Brainstorm a list of possible mentors
Step 6. Eliminate options that do not meet the "musts"	Evaluate each possible mentor against the "musts." If the candidate cannot fulfill them, do not consider him or her further
Step 7. Rate each option against "wants"	Compare how well each of the remaining options stacks up against your "wants." Assign a numeric rating (eg, 1–10) for each potential mentor to measure how well he or she measures up against each "want"
Step 8. Make the decision	Tally the numeric score to identify which of the candidates best meets your desired end result based on the criteria you established

this same group, 74.7% reported having a mentor but only 17.9% reported being "very satisfied" with their mentorship opportunities. Furthermore, Flint and colleagues found that orthopedic residents were most satisfied with mentoring when there was a formal program in place as well as if they selected their own mentor rather than having one assigned.[2] Mentorship has additionally been shown to be particularly important for minority and underrepresented groups in orthopedics, with women making up 13% of orthopedic surgery residents and minorities between 3% and 10% of orthopedic surgeons.[3,4] Oladeji and colleagues found that minorities were less likely to have multiple mentors and were more likely to be dissatisfied with the quality of their mentorship during residency, whereas women reported more often pursuing a mentor on their own.[4]

Selecting a Mentor

Appropriate selection and pairing of a mentor is critical to developing a 2-way relationship that will be rewarding for both the mentor and mentee. Pairing mentees and mentors with similar interests can be vital to the success of the relationship.[5] Self-selecting a mentor can allow for a more successful relationship over forced assignments. Taking the initiative to personally seek out a mentor with similar interests and definitions of success to the mentee has been shown to enhance the relationship.[5] A mentee should aim to select a mentor that has similar interests, they are comfortable asking questions to and they have the capability to have a high degree of contact. A mentee should look for a mentor that has accomplished specific goals that he or she would like to aim for in their career. Although having goals that align with each other's is important, selecting a mentor with specific differences that will challenge the mentee can allow for future growth. Finally, the mentee should take the time to meet with the mentor and assess compatibility to enhance the likelihood of success.

In "The Mentee's Guide: Making Mentoring Work for You," Zachary and Fischler propose a criteria-based decision making model that can be used for systematically identifying and selecting a mentor based on a step-wise progression of criteria (**Table 1**).[6]

Although not everyone will find such an approach necessary, the value of identifying the key qualities and attributes in a mentor and ensuring that those qualities and attributes align with the mentee's goals for the relationship cannot be overstated. In her mentorship series published in Forbes Magazine, Ashira Prossak states that there are 4 key things to look for in a mentor: compatibility (make sure you can work together), contrast (step outside your comfort zone and get different perspectives), expertise (which does not necessarily mean the most experienced or biggest title), and trust (which should go both ways).[7–9] Developing personal mission and career vision statements can help the mentee clarify, which attributes in a mentor will be most beneficial and which will align well with his/her goals. Clarifying these statements before the search for a mentor will help identify the key criteria in a mentor that will be most beneficial and best aligned with the mentee's. Above all, an honest appraisal of the primary needs of the mentee is paramount, as is an honest appraisal of what the mentor can offer.

Another key to finding the right mentor lies in defining the roles and expectations of the relationship. Does the mentee need an advocate for career advancement? Does the mentee need someone to provide honest, and perhaps negative, feedback? Someone to listen? Emotional support? Motivational support? Research expertise? Leadership advice? Guidance for work life balance? Or all of the above? Although the mentor/mentee relationship is certainly not limited to a single characteristic, the mentee should select a mentor whose strengths align with the role or roles that he/she most desires from the relationship.

In their Harvard Business Review article entitled "What Mentors Wish Their Mentees Knew", Vineet Chopra and Sanjay Saint clarify that mentorship can assume many shapes and roles.[10] The authors state that, at times, the mentee may need a coach to improved performance on a given issue (eg, preparing for a podium presentation). At other times, a sponsor is needed and can use their standing to leverage opportunities for the mentee to apply for committees, research projects, or selective memberships. Finally, some mentors can act as connectors that help the mentee establish or expand his/her professional network.[10] The mentor–mentee relationship is optimized when the optimal role that a mentor can play is aligned with the needs of the mentee.

In addition to defining the needs of the relationship, honestly assessing and discussing the limitations of the relationship is critical. Time constraints, geographic limitations, or even physical limitations can affect the mentor–mentee relationship and should be discussed openly, before or early in the relationship. Specifically, if the mentor is a direct supervisor, one should proceed with caution. If the mentor is the direct supervisor of the mentee, open communication, honest feedback, and authenticity may be compromised. Although most department chairs and division chiefs do engage in mentorship of those within their charge, the mentee may feel less opportunity to be completely open when discussing frustrations, long-term career plans, or struggles and challenges. Although the mentorship from a direct supervisor can be valuable, selecting a direct supervisor as the sole or primary mentor may be ill-advised.

It is important to recognize that most orthopedic surgeons have more than one mentor. It is extremely difficult, if not impossible, to find a mentor that excels in all areas, and meets all of the mentee's "needs" and "wants." Therefore, most orthopedic surgeons have multiple mentors. Although some overlap may occur, some mentors

Table 2
Unique roles/responsibilities of the mentee by level of orthopedic training

Mentee Level	Examples of Unique Roles/Responsibilities
Medical School	• Seek out a senior mentor in field of interest by directly reaching out/joining a formal mentorship program • Make time to meet/shadow/participate in research • Be engaged when present with mentor • Do a good job/be on time with all volunteered assignments
Residency	• Seek out a peer resident mentor to help guide through residency • Seek out an attending physician mentor to direct subspecialty/career decisions • Be smart about volunteering your time and follow through on commitments
Fellowship	• Determine what your goals are for fellowship year including clinical, educational, research, and practice-building and life • Seek out an attending mentor in your subspecialty to guide career decisions
Practice	• Seek out a colleague to be able to freely consult for clinical questions • Seek out a mentor(s) to help guide practice/personal life decisions • If continued research involvement is desired, partner with a clinician-researcher with similar interests

will excel in research mentorship, whereas others may provide more insight into practice building, some may be best suited to advocating for career advancement opportunities, whereas still others may be more suited to provide work/life balance mentorship. Roles and specific needs of mentors also evolve with different stages of training for the mentee (**Table 2**).[11] For example, the role of a mentor for a medical student may be more focused on giving the student means to explore their interests and providing access to pathways to be able to pursue a career in orthopedics. The role of a mentor for new attendings in practice is quite different. Often young surgeons need guidance on practice management, someone to ask clinical questions, and direction on how to best balance work and home responsibilities. There certainly is no limit to the number of mentors that one can have but searching for the "perfect mentor" that fills every role at the same time will undoubtedly prove to be a challenging endeavor.

Additionally, mentors may come and go. It is important for the mentor and mentee to continually engage in open and honest assessment of the relationship. If the relationship achieves its goals, one or both parties may decide to amicably bring the mentoring relationship to a close. It can be more challenging to end the relationship if one party feels that the relationship is falling short of the stated objectives. However, neither party will benefit if the relationship continues when unproductive or forced.

Finally, similar to all relationships, the mentor/mentee relationship will benefit if both parties take the time to get to know one another, invest in developing rapport, and proceed with mutual respect. It may take an investment of time and intentionality to deepen the personal connection between mentor and mentee but the investment will be well worth it and will not only ensure that the mentee has selected the right mentor but will serve as a good foundation for a productive mentoring relationship.

Responsibilities of the Mentee

It is imperative that the mentee realize that the mentor–mentee relationship is not a one-way street in which the mentor unilaterally provides knowledge and guidance. Expectations of being "spoon fed" information, advice, and opportunities will likely lead to frustration and lack of progress in the relationship. It is incumbent on the mentee to work diligently on the relationship, and several responsibilities fall to the mentee. If carried out appropriately, the relationship is more likely to be successful, meaningful, and productive.

First, the mentee should demonstrate dedication to his/her work. Whether it be clinical, research, leadership opportunities, or community involvement the mentor is much more likely to engage and provide impactful guidance when the mentee demonstrates commitment and dedication. If the mentee is simply "going through the motions" to satisfy a requirement, the mentor is less likely to invest significant time and effort. Exhibiting a strong commitment to the topic at hand is more likely to lead to buy in from the mentor.

The mentee should also be receptive to feedback. Avoid the temptation to become defensive or dismissive of negative feedback or constructive criticism. Although sometimes tough to hear, this type of advice and feedback can be invaluable. If developed properly, the mentor–mentee relationship offers a safe space for some of the best and most constructive feedback an orthopedic surgeon can receive—even if not always positive. If the mentee is not willing to accept honest feedback, the relationship will be compromised because the mentor will feel less likely to speak freely about his/her observations and expectations. Therefore, it is imperative that the mentee demonstrate a willingness to listen and receive this type of feedback, even if the advice is not implemented or the mentee ultimately disagrees. At the same time, the mentee should accept and appreciate positive feedback as well. At times, this can be challenging and the temptation for the mentee may think that the mentor is offering faint praise. Certainly, this can happen at times but if the mentee has carefully selected the right mentor, honest appraisals of positive performance and strengths should provide confidence and direction for the mentee. Again, an experienced mentor has experience and perspective that the mentee likely does not, and positive feedback should be accepted just as readily as constructive criticism or advice.

Finally, the mentee should approach each mentoring session willing to listen, learn, discern, and implement. There are times where the mentee will drive the conversation and may actually dominate the conversation. Talking through challenges and difficult scenarios with a mentor can provide clarity and organization of thought but ultimately the mentor–mentee relationship thrives because of 2-way flow of information. The mentee must be willing to listen and learn from the mentor. Ultimately, the mentor's expertise provides value to the mentee, and approaching the mentoring sessions with a willingness to listen and learn will ultimately provide more value to the mentee. However, the mentor must contemplate the lessons learned and advice received before implementation. Recognizing that not all information and recommendations are to be blindly followed, the mentee should take time to discern and accept or respectfully decline the recommendations from the mentor. Open and honest communication between the mentor and mentee after careful contemplation by the mentee can improve the value and deepen the bonds of the mentorship relationship, rather than blind acceptance or dismissing things out of hand.

Nicholas Pulos, MD, and Alexander Shin, MD, wrote about 3 distinct paths a mentee–mentor relationship can take, with the ideal path being one where the mentor and mentee grow to be colleagues and equals with an eventual role reversal between the 2 parties where the older surgeon can learn new techniques from the younger surgeon.[12] A second path is a quiet departure from the relationship allowing it to fizzle with distance and time. The final third path is the most challenging where the mentor will not allow for evolution of the relationship with role reversal with the mentee

Box 1
Tips for mentees

1. Respect Your Mentor's Time
   a. Arrive on time or early for meetings with your mentor. Arriving late not only wastes your mentor's time (which can be precious), it sends the message that you do not value the relationship as you should. If an issue arises and you will be late, communicate with your mentor.
   b. Schedule at mutually beneficial times and locations. Consider work and family schedules, time zone differences, and optimal duration of the meeting. Your mentor has many demands on his/her time, so take the time to find out the times, dates, locations, and types of meetings that work best for your mentor.

2. Clearly Communicate Expectations and Needs
   a. At the start of the mentor–mentee relationship, communicate with your mentor why you need him/her. What are your expectations and needs? Do you have specific short-term goals that you need help with, or are you looking for a career long mentor? What are your areas of need and concern? Let your mentor know with clear communication. (eg, I need to develop my career research plan; I would like advice on career planning; You have a successful practice and wonderful family life and I would like to emulate that)
   b. For mentoring sessions: have a plan for the meeting. The major error is to arrive at a meeting with your mentor without an agenda. This can be written or verbally communicated ahead of time, or at the start of the meeting. Avoid the pitfall of showing up to the mentoring session where both parties say, "what are we going to talk about today?" Having a planned topic or topics of discussion will optimize your time with your mentor and keep the discussion properly focused. Ideally, the agenda or plan is communicated to the mentor ahead of time so that he/she has time to think and prepare. If your meeting is purely social, that can be communicated as well.

3. Always have something on the calendar
   a. Avoid the temptation to end with "Let us talk again soon." Always have something on the calendar. A healthy relationship requires regular contact and communication. As the mentee, you can and should feel responsible for scheduling meetings. Take the initiative and always have something scheduled. At the end of the meeting, set expectations for when you would prefer to meet again. Do not wait for your mentor to reach out to you; be proactive and take the initiative at scheduling your meetings and communications.
   b. Maintain good communication with your mentor via phone calls, emails, texts, or in person visits. Regular communication will strengthen the relationship.

4. Be honest
   a. Be honest with yourself and your mentor about the relationship, what you need, and what your expectations are. If you are not getting what you need from the relationship, communicate honestly and respectfully with your mentor. If you receive advice that you disagree with, or decide not to act on, let your mentor know. This will ultimately help your mentor understand you and provide better mentorship.

5. Be prepared and direct
   a. As stated above, be prepared for your meetings with your mentor. Demonstrate your commitment to the relationship and let your mentor know you value them by preparing for your meetings.
   b. If you need something from your mentor, do not wait for them to read your mind or guess what you need. Be direct and communicate those needs clearly. If you have created a strong relationship with your mentor, you should not feel hesitant in letting him/her know your "asks," even if the mentor ultimately cannot comply.

6. Give feedback
   a. Just as it is important to receive feedback from your mentor, you should send feedback the other direction as well. If your mentor had a great idea that you implemented, let them know. If your mentor advocated for you, show appreciation. If your mentor could improve in certain areas, let him/her know that as well. Providing feedback to your

mentor ultimately helps clarify your evaluation of the relationship and guides your future mentorship experience with him/her.

Adapted from Chopra and Saint. What Mentors Wish Their Mentees Knew. Harvard Business Review. November 7, 2017.[10]

resulting in demise of the relationship. Continued growth for both the mentee and the mentor are necessary to continue to foster a healthy and beneficial relationship.

Optimizing the Mentee/Mentor Relationship: What Can the Mentee Do?

There are several "tips" that mentees can follow in order to optimize time with mentors and strengthen the relationship (**Box 1**). Ultimately, this can lead to a more productive and gratifying mentorship experience. As stated by Chopra and Saint: "Mentors are looking for closers: those that finish what they start. Ideal mentees...are enthusiastic, energetic, organized, and focused...and always behave with integrity."[10]

Ultimately, mentees should remember that they are the owners of their own professional development. Although mentors can help guide and facilitate goals and career paths, it is up to the mentee to drive the relationship, determine what is most important to them personally and professionally, and to take action toward goals.

SUMMARY

Mentorship in orthopedics is an important factor in career advancement and developing a well-rounded surgeon. The mentee plays a key role in creating and fostering this relationship. Self-selection of a mentor with similar interests often leads to a more successful relationship but should allow for some unique differences to foster personal growth. Attributes of successful mentees include willingness to initiate and engage in a relationship, honesty, open communication, being prepared, teachability, and being respectful of the mentor's time and experience. The needs and roles of a mentor for the mentee change with time, and it is advantageous for a mentee to have more than one mentor for different aspects and stages of their career and life. The mentee–mentor relationship should be a fulfilling one to both parties and allow for the mentee to reach their maximum potential both personally and professionally.

DISCLOSURE

The authors have no relevant disclosures.

REFERENCES

1. Hart RA, Eltorai A, Yanney K, et al. Update on mentorship in orthopaedic resident education. J Bone Joint Surg 2020;102(5):e20.
2. Flint JH, Jangir AA, Browner BD, et al. The value of mentorship in orthopaedic surgery resident education: the residents' perspective. J Bone Joint Surg Am 2009;91(4):1017e1022.
3. Oladeji LO, Ponce BA, Worley JR, et al. Mentorship in orthopedics: a national survey of orthopedic surgery residents. J Surg Educ 2018;75(6):1606–14. Epub 2018 Apr 25. PMID: 29685787.
4. Mulcahey MK, Waterman BR, Hart R, et al. The role of mentoring in the development of successful orthopaedic surgeons. J Am Acad Orthop Surg 2018;26(13): 463–71. PMID: 29847421.

5. Gofton W, Regehr G. Factors in optimizing the learning environment for surgical training. Clin Orthopaedics Relat Res August 2006;449:100–7.

6. Zachary L, Fischler L. The mentee's guide: making mentoring work for you. San Fransisco, CA: Jossey-Bass; 2009.

7. Prossak A. How to be a great mentee, ForbesWomen, Apr 27, 2018. Available at: https://www.forbes.com/sites/ashiraprossack1/2018/04/27/how-to-be-a-great-mentee/?sh=ea4dc25512b4. Accessed September, 2022.

8. Prossak A. 5 ways to get the most out of your mentor relationship, Forbeswomen, Apr 26, 2018. Available at: https://www.forbes.com/sites/ashiraprossack1/2018/04/26/5-ways-to-get-the-most-out-of-your-mentor-relationship/?sh=568983b17cf6. Accessed September, 2022.

9. Prossak A. 4 things to look for in a mentor, ForbesWomen, Apr 27, 2018. https://www.forbes.com/sites/ashiraprossack1/2018/04/27/4-things-to-look-for-in-a-mentor/?sh=5dbb197a2d47. Accessed Sept 2022.

10. Chopra V, Saint S. What mentors wish their mentees knew. Harv Bus Rev 2017.

11. Aiyer AA, Mody KS, Dib AG, et al. Medical student mentorship in orthopaedic surgery. J Am Acad Orthop Surg 2021;29(16):681–90. PMID: 34043604.

12. Pulos, Nicholas MD, Shin AY. Mentorship: perspectives through the eyes of the mentee and mentor. Tech Hand Upper Extremity Surg 2021;25 -(4):207.

Leadership

Leading Change in Health Care

Neil E. Grunberg, PhD[a],*, John E. McManigle, MD[a], Eric B. Schoomaker, MD, PhD[a], Erin S. Barry, MS[b]

KEYWORDS

- Change leadership • Health care • Individuals • TEAMS • Organizations

KEY POINTS

- Change leadership is essential in health care.
- Meaningful change in health care requires involvement of individuals and organizations.
- Several perspectives, models, and theories of change leadership can be applied to health care.
- The Leader-Follower Framework (LF2) can help guide leaders and followers to effect health-care changes.

The only constant in life is change.

—*Heraclitus (circa 500 bce)[1]*

INTRODUCTION

Change leadership focuses on leadership to initiate, support, and adapt to modifications, alterations, and new situations. Many different perspectives, models, theories, and steps to optimize change have been offered regarding change leadership. Based on a review of the literature and its variable use of language, we consider it important to provide the following definitions to guide the present article and to provide a basis for discussing change leadership within health care.

Leadership has been defined as "influence on individuals and groups by enhancing behaviors (actions), cognitions (perceptions, thoughts, and beliefs), and motivations (why we act and think as we do) to achieve goals that benefit the individuals and groups.",[2] p.2.

Change has been defined as "to make different, modify, or replace."[3]

Change Leadership has been defined as "ability *to influence and enthuse others*, through personal advocacy, vision and drive, and to access resources to build a solid

[a] Department of Military & Emergency Medicine, Uniformed Services University, 4301 Jones Bridge Road, Bethesda, MD 20814, USA; [b] Department of Anesthesiology, Uniformed Services University, 4301 Jones Bridge Road, Bethesda, MD, USA
* Corresponding author.
E-mail address: neil.grunberg@usuhs.edu

Clin Sports Med 42 (2023) 249–260
https://doi.org/10.1016/j.csm.2022.11.007
0278-5919/23/Published by Elsevier Inc.

sportsmed.theclinics.com

platform for change.",[4] p. 124 More recently, change leadership has been defined as the "ability *to influence and inspire action in others*, and respond with vision and agility during periods of growth, disruption or uncertainty to bring about the needed change."[5][*emphasis added*]

Although these definitions and concepts overlap, there are a few differences worth noting. Leadership, in general, involves influence that provides vision, inspires motivation, and encourages actions that bring people together. Change leadership, in particular, focuses on leadership to initiate, support, and adapt to modifications, alterations, and new situations. Several change leadership scholars and consultants have emphasized the role of the leader(s) to identify changes to be made and to influence followers to support and adapt to the changes. The current change leadership literature emphasizes influencing followers to help identify what to change; to prepare for and adapt to changes; and to make the changes necessary to optimize individual and organizational successes. It is essential for leaders and followers to recognize the need for change, especially in volatile, uncertain, complex, and ambiguous environments, as well as to overcome the inherent inertia of individuals, teams, and organizations to change. This recognition and acceptance is especially important when an organization has enjoyed success—the longer the period of success, the more challenging and potentially problematic to enact change.

Change Leadership in Health Care

Within health care, changes are constantly occurring. Efforts to improve health and health-care data fidelity and transparency have been especially important. These efforts have highlighted failures to protect patients from care-associated injuries and complications as well as suboptimal outcomes from an increasingly complex and balkanized system of care.[6] These changes include organizational and system structural changes, processes and practices, resources and personnel. Organizational changes are those such as adaptation to new patient records and billing systems, use of information technology and artificial intelligence, and best practice approaches to improve health and achieve optimal health-care outcomes while minimizing costs and maintaining patient safety and care. Changes in health care that focus on the people are changes such as improving collaboration, communication, and well-being among health-care team members (including health-care practitioners, administrators and policy-makers, patients, and patients' significant others); equitable treatment of all patients and colleagues; whole person care and prevention; diversity and inclusivity among health-care professionals; and reduction of health-care disparities and inequities.[7]

Leading change in health care certainly includes the organizational level, ranging from business, economic, and resource concerns to the people involved in delivering and receiving health care, yet it is important to remember that leading change in health care involves much more. Health-care change should consider personal, interpersonal, team, as well as organizational psychosocial levels. Personal health-care change leadership is important for health-care practitioners as well as patients to maximize well-being and to avoid burnout. Interpersonal health-care change leadership is relevant to every dyadic relationship, including practitioner with patient, practitioner with colleague, practitioner with patient's significant others. Team health-care change leadership is especially relevant to readers of this journal because teams include the health-care team and teams (eg, sports teams) as a group of beneficiaries of the health and health-care efforts. Organizational health care change is, of course, relevant to large groups, hospitals, institutions, systems, nations, and cultures. Because health-care settings often have high "change" (or turnover) of personnel, it is particularly important to consider how to lead health-care change in ways that will enhance performance and minimize disruptions or errors. No recent event has highlighted this better than the COVID-19 pandemic when nursing staffs in particular experienced high turnover with large numbers of itinerant nurses spending short periods in any one facility or system before moving to another community.[8]

This article briefly describes different leadership change models and concepts in the chronologic order in which they were proposed as a foundation for a discussion of how they can be applied to lead change in health care. Several of these models appeared in the business literature as either change management or change leadership models. Additionally, a couple models appeared in the psychology literature and the leadership literature. Each model is classified with regard to its emphasis either on "organizational change" or on "individual responses to change." It is noteworthy that organizational change *per se* was the focus of most models in the second half of the twentieth century literature, whereas individual responses to change have been the focus of most models in the twenty-first century literature. There is great value to consider and draw on these various models that offer different perspectives and approaches relevant to change in order to determine how to lead change in health care most effectively.

MAJOR CHANGE MODELS
Lewin's Change Management Model (1940s)—Organizational Change

Mathematical and social psychologist Kurt Lewin proposed a Change Management Model[9] that focused on organizational change and teams within the organization. It was simple to describe but not particularly easy to execute. The 3 stages of Lewin's Change Management Model are unfreeze, change, and refreeze. In other words, the first step is to identify systems, processes, practices, culture, and so forth that are currently in place in a given organization (ie, "frozen") and "unfreeze" them (ie, accept that they must be changed). The second step is to determine what should be changed and how those organizational elements need to be changed. The third step is to establish or "freeze" the new systems, processes, practices, culture. This approach offers a broad brush way of thinking about organizational changes and has been applied in some health-care settings.[10,11]

Plan-Do-Check-Act (1950s)—Organizational Change

Statistician and business consultant W. Edwards Deming developed the Deming Wheel or Control Cycle that includes 4 steps: Plan-Do-Check-Act (PDCA).[12] This PDCA model is an iterative process with the goal of achieving continuous change and improvement. Deming applied this approach to help rebuild Japanese businesses after World War II, and it became popular among US businesses and various organizations in the 1980s and 1990s. With regard to health care, the PDCA model was adopted by the Joint Commission for Healthcare Organizations (now The Joint Commission) as Continuous Quality Improvement.[13] The authors of the present article applied this method in the early 1990s at the Uniformed Services University of the Health Sciences to develop the USU Strategic Plan.

Kübler-Ross Change Curve (1969)—Individual Responses to Change

Elisabeth Kübler-Ross published *Death and Dying*[14] in which she proposed 5 psychological stages of grief: denial, anger, bargaining, depression, and acceptance. Kübler-Ross argued that these stages of grief should be accepted both by those experiencing them and by others to better understand people who are moving through these psychological stages. Some business leaders applied these stages to employees experiencing workplace change to help leaders optimally deal with their employees and for the employees to move through the stages to reach the stage of acceptance of the organizational changes.[15] This use of the Kübler-Ross Change Curve to help effect changes in businesses was unusual at the time because of its focus on individual responses of followers to change, rather than focusing on the organizational changes without consideration of individual employees' reactions to change.

McKinsey 7s Model (1970s)—Organizational Change

Thomas J. Peters and Robert H. Waterman at management consulting firm, McKinsey & Company, developed the 7s model to evaluate how parts of an organization work together. They identified 7 elements of organizations categorized into hard and soft elements. The hard elements (ie, easiest to identify and control) are strategy, structure, and system. The soft elements (ie, that are more subjective and more difficult to change) are shared values, staff, style, and skills.[16] They proposed that these 7 elements are interconnected and that changing one affects all of the other elements. Therefore, companies and organizations that effect change should be aware of all of these 7 elements to align and balance the changes within parts of the larger organization.

Stages of Change Model (Late 1970s)—Individual Responses to Change

Psychologists James Prochaska and Carlo DiClemente proposed a Stages of Change Model (aka the Transtheoretical Model [TTM]) to focus on individual and intentional change of health-related behaviors (eg, abstain from tobacco use, alter diet, and exercise).[17] TTM was *not* proposed or applied to organizational change or to individual responses to organizational changes. However, TTM is a valuable model to help leaders and followers respond to change in organizations as well as in their personal lives. TTM assumes that people do not change behaviors quickly and decisively. Rather, change in behavior occurs through a purposeful, cyclical process that involves 6 stages of change: precontemplation, contemplation, preparation, action, maintenance, and termination. In the *precontemplation* stage, people do not intend to take action in the foreseeable future (ie, within the next 6 months). In the *contemplation* stage, people intend to start the healthy behavior in the foreseeable future (ie, within the next 6 months). In the *preparation* (or *determination*) stage, people are ready to take action within the next 30 days. In the *action* stage, people have recently changed their behavior (ie, within the last 6 months), and they intend to persist with that behavior change. In the *maintenance* stage, people have sustained their behavior change (ie, more than 6 months), intend to maintain the behavior change, and work to prevent relapse to earlier stages and unwanted behavior. In the *termination* stage, people have established the new behavior change and have no desire to return to the previous behaviors.

Change Commitment Curve (1982)—Individual Responses to Change

Conner and Patterson developed the "Change Commitment Curve" to describe individual responses to organizational changes over time.[18] This model identifies 3 phases that reflect degree of support individuals have for new mindsets or behaviors: preparation, acceptance, and commitment. The *preparation* phase includes contact and awareness—people become aware of the change and why it is needed. The *acceptance* phase includes understanding and positive perception—team members understand what is expected of them with the change. The *commitment* phase includes adoption, institutionalization, and internalization—the change has occurred and team members must make it a part of their lives.

Bridges Transition Model (1991)—Individual Responses to Change

William Bridges created the Bridges Transition Model as a people-centered approach to change management based on the Kübler-Ross Change Curve.[19] According to the Bridges Transition Model, the key to successful change management depends on whether and how individuals let go of the old and accept the change. According to this model, there are 3 stages that occur when people transition to change: (1) Ending, losing, and letting go; (2) Neutral zone: in which team members adapt to the change(s); (3) New beginnings when changes are accepted.

Conner Model (1992)—Individual Responses to Change

Daryl R. Connor built on the Change Commitment Curve in his book.[20] Conner thinks that people will resist change, so senior managers/leaders should prepare answers for followers to questions that address such issues as: what was wrong with the way things were done before; what do the changes mean for me; and what is going to happen now? Conner further held that we now live in an era of perpetual change and that we need to expect more change. He argues that we should not focus on making people feel comfortable during a major change. Instead, leaders should help people adjust to change and to succeed in the context of the change(s). Connor suggests that organizational leaders need to manage the amount of change that their followers experience and to keep it within tolerance levels that they can handle. In addition, Connor emphasizes the need for change leaders to recognize and address the cycle of emotions people experience with change, similar to the Bridges Transition Model and Kübler-Ross grief cycle.[20,21]

Kotter's 8-Step Change Model (1996)—Organizational Change

John Kotter's 8-step change model is, perhaps, the most highly cited business change model.[22–24] Similar to the emphasis in the twentieth century, Kotter's approach focuses on organizational change initiated by managers and leaders and also getting followers to buy-in to the organizational changes. According to Kotter, there are 8 steps to successful change to which leaders should attend: (1) Create a sense of urgency; (2) Build a guiding coalition; (3) Form a strategic vision and initiatives; (4) Enlist a volunteer army; (5) Enable action by removing barriers; (6) Generate short-term wins; (7) Sustain acceleration; and (8) Institute change. It is noteworthy that Kotter emphasizes the role of the leader or manager to initiate and monitor every step of the change process. This emphasis on the role of the leader differs from most other modern approaches to effective change leadership.

Three C's of Change Leadership (2000)—Individual Responses to Change

Three C's of change leadership were emphasized that focus on relationships and involvement of leaders and followers—communicate, collaborate, and commit.[25,26] Identification of these 3 C actions highlights a view of change leadership as an activity that involves all members of the team rather than depending on particular positions, responsibilities, and roles.

Adaptation to Effect Change Leadership (2001)—Individual Responses to Change

According to Heifetz and Laurie, there are 2 key points with regard to leading change successfully that require involvement and change among leaders and followers: (1) Individuals must change themselves as well as change their organizations, and (2)

Adaptive challenges require leaders and followers to learn and apply new ways to think about and do their work.[27] These authors underscore the difficulties posed by challenging situations as well as the importance that all members of the team work to change themselves and their organizations to optimize likelihood of effective adaptation and change.

Action Logic and Change (2005)—Individual Responses to Change

Rooke and Torbett[28] emphasize the importance of leaders understanding and changing/developing their "action logic" so that their organizations can transform/change as needed. According to these authors, there are 7 developmental action "logics" or ways of thinking and approaching situations. These 7 different action logics have been labeled as follows: opportunist, diplomat, expert, achiever, individualist, strategist, or alchemist. Although these authors focus on self-awareness and development of leaders, understanding and developing action logic can help leaders and followers adapt to and accept change.

ADKAR Model (2006)—Individual Responses to Change

Jeffery Hiatt focused on establishing buy-in and individual responses to change of followers to achieve successful organizational change.[29] ADKAR is an acronym for the 5 steps that followers need to embrace for organizational change to be accomplished. The 5 steps are as follows: (1) *Awareness* of the need to change, (2) *Desire* to change and buy-in, (3) *Knowledge* to help prepare for change, (4) *Ability to* perform effectively after the change, and (5) *Reinforcement* to sustain the change.

Generative Change Agent Development Programs (2008)—Individual Responses to Change

Alain Gautier wrote about Generative Change Agent Development (GCAD) programs[30] and McIntosh's Integral Consciousness and the Future of Evolution[31] that develop "integral approaches" that include "interior" and "exterior" dimensions of individual and collective (group and organizational) development to allow deep and sustainable change. "Interior" dimensions refer to aspects of individuals and groups/organizations, such as intention, worldview, purpose, vision, values, and cultural norms. "Exterior" dimensions refer to aspects of individuals and groups/organizations, such as behaviors, organizational structures, and processes.

Adaptive Leadership for Changing Organizations (2009)—Individual Responses to Change

Heifetz, Grashow, and Linsky built on earlier study by Heifetz and Laurie[27] to emphasize the importance of leaders themselves adapting and changing to allow their organizations to change.[32] These authors continue to include the need for all individuals, leaders, and followers, to change in parallel with organizational changes. However, this 2009 version of Heifetz and colleagues focuses on the critical importance of leaders themselves changing.

7 Dynamics of Change (Circa 2010)—Individual Responses to Change

According to Blanchard, change is inevitable and most people hate change.[33] Blanchard identified 7 dynamics of change that are predictable patterns of how most people deal with change. He argued that understanding and addressing these 7 dynamics of change, especially among followers, are necessary to enact change. The 7 dynamics of change are that people: (1) Feel awkward, ill-at-ease, self-conscious, or fearful about change; (2) Focus on what they have to give up; (3) Feel alone, even if everyone else is going through the same change; (4) Can handle only so much change; (5) Are at different levels of readiness for change; (6) Are concerned that they do not have enough resources to cope with the change; and (7) Revert to their old behaviors if given the opportunity.

Innovative Leadership to Transform Organizations (2013)—Organizational and Individual Responses to Change

According to Metcalf, innovative leadership is needed to lead organizational change.[34] Innovative leadership includes understanding and developing 5 key elements:

1. Leader type;
2. Developmental perspective;
3. Resilience;
4. Situational analysis; and
5. Leadership behaviors.

Innovative leadership is based on the recognition that 4 dimensions exist and influence interactive experiences: intention, behavior, culture, and systems. The process steps of innovative leadership are create a vision and sense of urgency, recruit and build team, analyze situations and strengths, plan journey, communicate, implement and measure, and embed transformation. When working to transform/change an organization, Metcalf encourages self-monitoring and use of change assessment instruments. Metcalf emphasizes using communication to support organizational change and help followers move up the Change Commitment Curve.

Leader-Follower Framework (LF2) (2018)—from Individual Responses to Change to Dyads, Teams, Organizations

Grunberg and colleagues[2,35] developed a conceptual framework of leadership based on a comprehensive review of leadership principles, models, and types. This framework includes 4 "C" elements—character, competence, context, communication—that operate across 4 levels of psychosocial interaction—personal, interpersonal, team, and organizational (PITO).[36] Barry and colleagues[37] extended this conceptual framework to the development of followers as well as leaders.

Character (Who the leader and followers are) refers to physical and psychological aspects of the individual. Character includes physical characteristics, appearance, demographics, attributes, personality, attitudes, beliefs, values honesty, integrity, trustworthiness, reliability, responsibility, and moral compass. Effective leaders and followers develop Character in positive ways, adapting to situations, learning and changing to meet new challenges and situations more effectively and efficiently, and adjusting to the demands of situations, resources available, and people involved.

Competence (What the leader and followers know and do) refers to role-specific knowledge and skills and to general (or transcendent) leadership knowledge and skills, including critical thinking, decision-making, problem-solving, futures thinking, motivating others, conflict resolution, emotional intelligence (EQ), and ability to adapt to change.

Context (When and Where leadership and followership occur) includes physical, psychological, social, and cultural environments and situations. Context also includes effects of physical and mental stress that alter judgment, perception, and performance of leadership and followership competence. Change, for individuals and organizations, present uncertainty and challenges that can be particularly stressful.

Communication (How leaders and followers interact) includes sending and receiving information, verbally and nonverbally. Leaders and followers are engaged in a relationship requiring trust, mutual respect, understanding, and sharing information. Verbal and nonverbal communication must be consistent with each other. It is important to practice effective sending and receiving communication skills and to be aware of perceptions and responses of senders and receivers, especially when dealing with change.

Personal refers to the individual leader or follower, especially elements of self-reflection and self-knowledge.

Interpersonal refers to dyadic relationships and interactions between the leader and followers, including members of the health care team as well as patients and their significant others.

Team refers to a small group of people with complementary skills who are mutually committed to common goals. Health-care teams include the various professionals who deliver health care as well as patients and their significant others.

Organizational refers to large groups, institutions, and systems.

LEADER-FOLLOWER FRAMEWORK (LF2) AND "CHANGE LEADERSHIP"

The Leader-Follower Framework can be used to guide leaders and followers when confronted with change on all psychosocial levels—personal, interpersonal, team, and organizational. Awareness of the 4 elements at each of the 4 psychosocial levels is relevant to effect and to accept health-care changes among people (including all health-care staff, patients, and people in patients' lives) within systems, cultures, and organizations relevant to health care.

On the *personal* level, health-care professionals experience profound changes in their roles, responsibilities, knowledge, and skills throughout their careers. For example, physicians must adapt to marked changes as they transition from premedical students to medical students to interns (postgraduate year [PGY]-1) to residents (PGY-2 and higher) to experienced physicians to various administrative, managerial, and leadership roles.

- Personal Character change requires health-care practitioners to be aware of and accept their own development and changes in roles, responsibilities, knowledge, skills, and attitudes (KSAs; ie, internal self-awareness). They also need to be aware of changes in how they are perceived by colleagues, patients, and patients' significant others (ie, external self-awareness) based on their role, responsibilities, demographics (eg, age), and apparent expertise. Intelligence, measured most often by IQ, is an element of character; although high cognitive intelligence is valuable, it is not easily changed—if at all—whereas EQ, a Personal Competence, is even more valuable and mutable. Many health-care practitioners experience "imposter syndrome" because they rapidly progress in roles and responsibilities, and they need to establish relationships with trusted colleagues who can provide advice, counsel, and collaboration.
- Personal Competence changes occur for health-care professionals because they experience marked and relatively rapid changes in role-specific KSAs with experience, education, training as well as changes in transcendent leadership KSAs (eg, critical thinking, problem-solving, decision-making, EQ, and conflict resolution).
- Personal Context also is ever-changing, including changes in "internal context" (eg, tiredness, exhaustion, burn-out) and "external context" (eg, physical, psychosocial, cultural settings in which health-care professionals work and spend nonwork time).
- Personal Communication change occurs because health-care professionals develop ways in which they take in and record information.

On the *interpersonal* psychosocial level, health-care professionals experience changes resulting from interactions with different individuals and from changes in one's role, responsibility, and authority.

- Interpersonal character dyadic changes depend on the others with whom we interact (eg, patients, supervisor, colleague, and subordinate).
- Interpersonal competence changes are based on the role-specific and transcendent competence of those with whom we interact, including the extent of understanding each other's motivations (ie, social intelligence).
- Interpersonal context changes in relationships with other individuals are based on each individual's roles, responsibilities, demands, stress, and relationships (eg, congenial and respectful, cooperative, or competitive).
- Interpersonal communication changes are based on the abilities and willingness of each individual to send and receive with the goal of achieving mutual understanding or not.

On the *team* level, changes result from changes of membership on a health-care team and one's role with teams of colleagues and patients.

- Team character changes are based on the values, mission, make up, cohesiveness, and morale of a team (including health-care teams and athletic or other teams)
- Team competence changes depend on the role-specific and transcendent competencies of the members of the team.
- Team context changes depend on relationships among team members and the situations and environments within which the teams perform.
- Team communication changes depend on the abilities, goals, communication styles, and relationships among team members.

On the *organizational* level, changes result from organizational changes in mission, priorities, needs, resources, culture, and so on.

- Organizational character changes with the mission, values, needs, goals, and style of an organization/system.
- Organizational competence changes with the role-specific and transcendent competencies of the organization/system as a whole.
- Organizational context changes depending on the demands, expectations, resources (including time, personnel, space, funds, and equipment) of the organizations/systems.
- Organizational communication changes are based on approaches, technology, and styles of communication within organizations/systems.

BRINGING IT ALL TOGETHER

Leading health-care change is critical and challenging. As with any important multidimensional human endeavor, attention to both the changing organization—whether a sports, medical, or military team, an academic institution, a business or service industry, nonprofit or governmental unit—and the individuals who comprise, manage, and lead the organization must be addressed. Many models have been proposed relevant to change that can be drawn on to help guide successful health-care change for organizations and individuals. They share many overlapping elements and principal foci. The key take-away messages from the models discussed in this article that focus on organizational change can be summed up as follows:

- Change the organization (Lewin's Change Management Model; Deming's PDCA).
- Consider elements to change the organization (McKinsey 7s model).
- Organization change is necessary and followers must get involved to change organizations (Kotter's 8-step change model).

The key take-away messages from the models discussed in this article that focus on individual responses to change can be summed up as follows:

- Recognize the challenges for people to change (Kübler-Ross Change Curve, Bridges Transition Model, Conner Model, and 7 Dynamics of Change).
- Recognize and encourage stages of change for leaders and followers (TTM, Change Commitment Curve, Action Logic, and GCAD).
- Engage and develop leaders and followers to enact change (Three C's of Change Leadership, Breakthrough Leadership, ADKAR, Adaptive Leadership, Innovative Leadership, and Leader-Follower Framework).

This article began with a quote from an Ancient Greek philosopher. It, therefore, seems fitting to close with reference to a Greek myth...but with an alternative interpretation. In the myth of Sisyphus, the wretched soul who must roll an immense bolder up a hill only to have it roll back to the base so that Sisyphus must repeat this seemingly pointless task for eternity. We suggest that Sisyphus' task is not pointless. Instead, it represents relentless and dedicated persistence that is required to accept and endlessly pursue and lead change. Health care can only be improved if we embrace the philosophy and actions of continuous effort with the goal of positive change.

DISCLOSURE

The authors do not have any commercial or financial conflicts of interest.

FUNDING

No funding was provided for this article.

DISCLAIMER

The opinions and assertions contained herein are the sole ones of the authors and are not to be construed as reflecting the views of the Uniformed Services University or the Department of Defense.

REFERENCES

1. Arapahoe T. "The only constant in life is change." - Heraclitus. Available at: https://arapahoelibraries.org/blogs/post/the-only-constant-in-life-is-change-heraclitus/#:~:text=One%20constant%20since%20the%20beginning,in%20control%20of%20our%20lives. Accessed June 25, 2022.
2. Grunberg NE, Barry ES, Callahan C, et al. A conceptual framework for leader and leadership education and development. Int J Leadersh Education 2018;1–7. https://doi.org/10.1080/13603124.2018.1492026.
3. Meriam-Webster. Change. In Merriam-Webster.com dictionary. Available at: https://www.merriam-webster.com/dictionary/change. Accessed June 1, 2022.
4. Higgs M, Rowland D. Building change leadership capability:'The quest for change competence'. J Change Manag 2000;1(2):116–30.

5. Akpoveta YR. Change Leadership Defined - No Longer for a Select Few. Change Leadersh 2019;2019. Available at: https://thechangeleadership.com/change-leadership-defined/#:~:text=Change%20Leadership%20is%20the%20ability%20to%20influence%20and%20inspire%20action,bring%20about%20the%20needed%20change. Accessed June 24, 2022.

6. Baker A. Crossing the quality chasm: a new health system for the 21st century, vol. 323. London, England, UK: British Medical Journal Publishing Group; 2001.

7. Loria K. The Future of Healthcare Leadership. Manag Healthc Executive 2019; 29(9). Available at: https://www.managedhealthcareexecutive.com/view/future-healthcare-leadership. Accessed June 24, 2022.

8. CareContent. Modern Healthcare's Next Up. How to prepare for a change in leadership with Lisa Spengler. 2021. Available at: https://www.modernhealthcare.com/labor/surviving-transitions-how-prepare-change-leadership-lisa-spengler.

9. Lucid Content Team. 7 Fundamental Change Management Models. Lucidchart. n.d. Available at: https://www.lucidchart.com/blog/7-fundamental-change-management-models#lewinmodel. Accessed June 1, 2022.

10. Šuc J, Prokosch H-U, Ganslandt T. Applicability of Lewin s change management model in a hospital setting. Methods Inf Med 2009;48(05):419–28.

11. Abd El-Shafy I, Zapke J, Sargeant D, et al. Decreased pediatric trauma length of stay and improved disposition with implementation of Lewin's change model. J Trauma Nurs JTN 2019;26(2):84–8.

12. The W. Edwards deming institute. PDSA cycle. Available at: https://deming.org/explore/pdsa/. Accessed June 1, 2022.

13. O'Leary DS, O'Leary MR. From quality assurance to quality improvement: the Joint Commission on Accreditation of Healthcare Organizations and emergency care. Emerg Med Clin North Am 1992;10(3):477–92.

14. Kübler-Ross E. On death and dying. New York, NY: MacMillian Company; 1969.

15. Rashford NS, Coghlan D. Phases and levels of organisational change. J Managerial Psychol 1989.

16. McKinsey JO. 7S model. strategic management insight. 2022. 2022. Available at: https://strategicmanagementinsight.com/tools/mckinsey-7s-model-framework/. Accessed June 1, 2022.

17. Behavioral Change Models. The transtheoretical model (stages of change). Available at: https://sphweb.bumc.bu.edu/otlt/mph-modules/sb/behavioralchange theories/behavioralchangetheories6.html. Accessed June 1, 2022.

18. Collaboratory. Theor into pract: the commitment curve. Available at: https://cecollaboratory.com/research-commitment-curve/. Accessed June 1, 2022.

19. Bridges W. Managing transitions: making the most of change. New York, NY: Perseus Books; 1991.

20. Conner DR. Managing at the speed of change: how resilient managers succeed and prosper where others fail. New York, NY: Random House; 1993.

21. Conner DR. Managing at the speed of change: The dos and don't of ongoing turbulence. Available at: https://www.strategies-for-managing-change.com/daryl-conner.html. Accessed June 1, 2022.

22. Kotter. The 8 steps for leading change. Available at: https://www.kotterinc.com/methodology/8-steps/. Accessed June 1, 2022.

23. Kotter JP. Leadership change. Boston: Harvard Business School Press; 1996.

24. Kotter JP. Leading change. Boston, MA: Harvard Business Press; 2012.

25. Hole G. The 3 C's of change leadership. Management Philosopher 2020;2020. Available at: https://www.dr-glennhole.org/the-3-cs-of-change-leadership/. Accessed June 1, 2022.

26. Leading Effectively Staff. How to be a successful change leader. center for creative leadership. Available at: https://www.ccl.org/articles/leading-effectively-articles/successful-change-leader/. Accessed June 1, 2022.

27. Heifetz RA, Laurie DL. The work of leadership. Harv business Rev 2001;75: 124–34.

28. Rooke D, Torbert WR. Seven Transformations of Leadership. Harvard Business Review; 2005. April 2005. Available at: https://hbr.org/2005/04/seven-transformations-of-leadership. Accessed June 1, 2022.

29. Hiatt J. ADKAR: a model for change in business, government, and our community. Prosci 2006.

30. Gautier A. Developing generative change leaders across sectors: an exploration of integral approaches. integral leadership review; 2008. Available at: https://integralleadershipreview.com/5061-feature-article-developing-generative-change-leaders-across-sectors-an-exploration-of-integral-approaches/. Accessed June 1, 2022.

31. McIntosh S. Integral consciousness and the future of evolution. St. Paul, MN: Paragon House; 2007.

32. Heifetz R, Grashow A, Linsky M. The practice of adaptive leadership: tools and tactics for changing your organization and the world. Boston, MA: Harvard Business Press; 2009.

33. Blanchard K. Seven dynamics of change. your better business content. Available at: https://betterbusinesscontent.com/product/seven-dynamics-change/. Accessed June 1, 2022.

34. Metcalf M. Innovative leaders guide to transforming organizations. Integral Publishers 2013.

35. Callahan CW, Grunberg NE. Military medical leadership. In: O'Connor FG, Schoomaker EB, Smith DC, editors. Fundamentals Mil Med. San Antonio, TX: Borden Institute; 2019. p. 51–66.

36. Price PA. Genesis and evolution of the united states air force academy's officer development system. DTIC Document. Available at: http://www.dtic.mil/dtic/tr/fulltext/u2/a428315.pdf. Accessed June 8, 2015.

37. Barry ES, Grunberg NE. A conceptual framework to guide leader and follower education, development, and assessment. J Leadersh Account Ethics 2020;17(1): 127–34.

Personal Growth and Emotional Intelligence
Foundational Skills for the Leader

Bobbie Ann Adair White, EdD, MA[a],*,
Joann Farrell Quinn, PhD, MBA[b]

KEYWORDS

- Emotional intelligence • Empathy • Professional development
- Conflict management • Leadership

KEY POINTS

- Emotional intelligence (EI) can be improved and enhanced.
- Physicians with EI make better leaders and doctors.
- Empathy and conflict management skills can be improved to influence personal and professional relationships.

INTRODUCTION

Take a minute to consider how an individual who lacks emotional intelligence (EI) shows up in the world. For example, the surgeon who upsets everyone with their tone or approach. This behavior is often diagnosed as a professionalism issue but instead it is often an issue with EI. Maybe the individual does not understand how their tone is perceived, maybe they do not manage their emotions well when in a stressful situation, or maybe they are incapable of understanding others' perceptions of their actions. No matter the diagnosis of that situation, EI or lack thereof most likely played a role. Emotional and social competencies make up what is termed EI and are the overriding difference in most contexts that require interaction including leadership, and relationships (personal and work). The goal of this article is highlight foundational EI skills through the lens of personal growth. Thus, the article starts with background, definitions, and historic components of EI, followed by information on core EI skills or components for personal growth, and finally, summary sections about professional development.

---

[a] MGH (Massachusetts General Hospital) Institute of Health Professions, Charlestown Navy Yard, 36 1st Avenue, Boston, MA 02129, USA; [b] University of South Florida, Morsani College of Medicine, Muma College of Business, 560 Channelside Drive MDD 54, Tampa, FL 33602, USA
* Corresponding author.
E-mail address: Bwhite2@mghihp.edu

Clin Sports Med 42 (2023) 261–267
https://doi.org/10.1016/j.csm.2022.11.008
0278-5919/23/© 2022 Elsevier Inc. All rights reserved.
sportsmed.theclinics.com

BACKGROUND

EI is the ability to have insight about yourself as well as others and the ability to manage your behavior and relationships. EI has been explored from a variety of perspectives and falls into 3 streams: stream 1—abilities, stream 2—traits, and stream 3—mixed models. Stream 1 includes inventories or measures for abilities, such as the Mayer Salovey Caruso EI Test[1]; stream 2 includes self-report measures of traits[2]; and stream 3 includes competency measures, including the Bar-On EQ-i (2004)[3] and Boyatzis and Goleman's (2007)[4] Emotional and Social Competency Inventory. Each stream explores EI from a different perspective but they all recognize the importance of understanding the self and regulating or managing behavior effectively, especially during particularly emotional moments.

The foundational competencies of EI provide an understanding of ourselves, an ability to manage our behavior, insight into others, and the capacity to manage our relationships well (**Table 1**). The resulting behaviors of these competencies have proven to be essential for individual and organizational effectiveness.

EI has gained increasing interest during the past couple of decades. First as a complement to standard intelligence and now as a separate necessity. The application of these skills is becoming universal, transitioning from being something seen as important for business leaders, to something that is important for everyone. Medical education and hospital medicine have also started to see the importance of EI or "human factors" with mandatory curriculum and accreditation requirements such as nontechnical skills for surgeons (NOTSS), professionalism curriculum, and Accreditation Council for Graduate Medical Education (ACGME) requirements.[5–7] Take notice that professionalism and NOTSS do not include EI in their vocabulary; however, if you inspect their content, both require EI. More recently, leaders who study EI in medicine oversaw article submissions and editorialized the collection, identifying baseline information about EI in medicine.[8] Interestingly, surgery has started to incorporate EI in their education and research.[9–12] It is often the nontechnical skills, such as EI competencies that create problems later when physicians struggle beyond the technical aspects of the role,[13] and in leadership roles, these skills are even more essential as the effects of lacking them are amplified.

An understanding of our emotions and the ability to manage ourselves is a prerequisite to interpersonal skills. These skills are core to functioning in both personal and professional life. More especially, these skills are key to navigating the nuances of medical practice; awareness and management of self and others are daily requirements because physicians work with ad hoc and long-term teams. Those who are unable to manage themselves experience more difficulty in interpersonal relationships and even disciplinary actions.

Core Emotional Intelligence Skills for Personal Growth

Empathy and communication skills

A core aspect of EI is empathy. In fact, some theorists have chosen to make it a fifth and separate domain to EI. However, many think it is embedded in the simplified

Table 1	
Domain of emotional intelligence	
Self-awareness—naming and understanding our emotions	Social-awareness—insight into others' emotions and affect
Self-management—managing our behavior and responses	Relationship-management—ability to facilitation positive relationships

model with only 4 domains. Empathy is the ability to connect with others. The word empathy has been used for over a century,[14] yet there are many definitions and understandings by different researchers. One study uncovered 43 definitions for empathy.[15] The definition that most closely falls within our understanding of how empathy is operationalized in terms of a competency is feeling *as* another, which differs from sympathy in feeling *for* another.[16]

The literature is clear from all streams, that EI has a potential impact on affect and therefore job performance.[17] Engaging empathy provides an opportunity to connect with others and connection is what enhances well-being and belonging. Additionally, empathy can be improved with intervention.[18] Thus, the empathy slip (when trainees' empathy reduces as training progresses) previously found in medical training can be combatted and instead empathy can be enhanced through interventions. If empathy is intentionally enhanced, then physicians will have better job performance and relationships.

To emote and connect, one must have effective communication skills. Communication is defined by Merriam-Webster as "a process by which information is exchanged between individuals through a common system of symbols, signs, or behavior." An important aspect of this definition is "information is exchanged" because often people perceive communication only as the telling or listening aspect. Instead, communication should be a dialog. People want to feel heard, and this includes patients.[19] In medicine communication can build relationships and relationships can help heal, coupling those together enables relationship-based communication, enhancing trust and patient health.[20]

Empathy and communication are skills that are unextractable from not just the doctor–patient relationship but are just as important for interacting with colleagues and serving as a leader. Both skills are core to EI and literature has shown both to be influenced by interventions and education. To learn more about empathy and communication, consider investigating some of the citations as well as the Academy of Professionalism in Healthcare and the Academy of Communication[21] in Healthcare; both organizations highlight cutting-edge research in these areas.

Conflict management

Conflict management is a core competency of EI and falls under the domain of relationship management.[22] However, conflict management in action requires every single domain of EI. An individual must be self-aware, which will enable them to manage their own emotions and reactions in the situation; they must also be aware of and read their colleagues' emotions and responses; and finally they must manage the relationship to ensure they are strengthening the team through collaboration. Lopes and colleagues (2011)[23] looked at conflict management and confirmed the importance of being able to identify emotional states of the individual and others', to effectively respond in a conflict.

Conflict is inevitable in all aspects of life, and medicine is no exception. Within many cultures both within and outside of the United States, conflict is perceived as negative, and people forget the positive components of conflict. If conflict is addressed in a positive way, it can lead to change, collaboration, and growth. However, if conflict is not addressed in a healthy way, it can lead to negative outcomes such as avoidant or toxic cultures and minimize psychological safety. To ensure a growth culture, it is important to properly manage and address conflict because unaddressed conflict becomes recurring conflict.

When managing conflict, it is important to identify the type(s) of conflict occurring to be sure all aspects of the conflict are addressed. If only one aspect of the conflict is addressed, then the remaining aspects will recur. According to Greer and colleagues (2012),[24] there are 3 primary types of conflict in medical teams: relationship, task, and process. Each conflict can include one or more of these types. For example, if there is a conflict between a doctor and a nurse about a particular order (ie, how often to move the patient after operation), it is important to identify the type of conflict. Is the conflict an existing relationship issue, meaning do the pair have a history of not getting along or disagreeing. If the relationship is not the issue, then is it a task issue, something that can be fixed more immediately, or is it a process issue, something that will require a change in process or protocol within the hospital. Often, conflict includes more than one type, yet individuals only address the easiest component, the task at hand. This is most often the quickest way to move forward; however, if the relationship or process issue is not addressed, then the next time this pair works together, issues will resurface. Not managing all types of conflict in a situation ensures recurrence and ultimately can lead to a toxic or avoidant culture.

From these authors' experience, one of the top reported conflicts or issues in medical teams and medical education settings is disrespect. People not feeling respected in their expertise, not feeling respected as a team member, or not feeling respected as an individual. This feeling of disrespect can often be a misunderstanding but it is a misunderstanding that would occur far less if relationship management was a priority as relationships encourage positive assumptions rather than negative ones. When it comes to difficult conversations, one of the best things you can do is build rapport and relationships before those conversations need to happen. Rapport and relationships are based on human connection, and that connection allows the other person to see a multidimensional person rather than a one-dimensional adversary, so empathy is given, and positive assumptions are made rather than negative assumptions. Thus, in most cases, putting the relationship first with relationship-based communication will build a stronger foundation for the team and for navigating difficult conversations.

Burnout

It is well established that medicine is a stressful vocation and one that leads to a high burnout rate.[25] Burnout in medicine has been defined as a "state of mental exhaustion caused by the doctor's professional life."[26] With burnout being a hot topic, it continues to be extensively studied. Boyatzis and McKee (2005)[27] identified leading with EI as a way to reduce burnout. Leading with EI ensures collaboration and connection within teams.[28] Additionally, emotional and social competencies enable an individual's resilience, lessening the influence of factors that lead to burnout.

Having the ability to reflect and recognize what emotions are affecting us allows the opportunity to attempt to respond appropriately, instead of reacting without thinking. Burnout can have many contributing factors including internal and external factors. Identifying internal and external factors and emotions can help diagnose situations and guide how to respond and react to shape mindset and work culture.

Leadership

Although health-care organizations have been led by physicians since the beginning of organized medicine, often physicians end up in leadership roles without adequate training in the basic skills and competencies needed to lead well. Physicians and trainees share that they would like more training in leadership. Physicians think that their primary role is within their area of clinical expertise, and leadership is an added responsibility, leading them to not fully identify as a leader,[29] which is not surprising because anecdotally these authors have noticed many, if not most, medical students do not identify as leaders. When starting leadership courses with these populations, the first step is helping them identify as a leader, and ultimately helping them see the importance of leadership training.

As leadership becomes more popular in medicine, so do leadership education programs. Despite the growth of leadership education programs, student competency or behavior change have not resulted.[30] A leadership framework that has had successful outcomes is resonant leadership, which can be used as an educational framework. Leading with EI has the positive effects of all aspects listed thus far including excellent relationship management, helping to reduce burnout, and the ability to build trust in teams (White and colleagues 2019). EI was found to be a key aspect of what took a good leader to a great leader.[22]

DISCUSSION

EI as a concept is catching on in medicine.[5] Unfortunately, a stigma remains around "soft skills," which has required authors to not directly use the EI term in titles. For example, these authors published a leadership text about leading with EI but were encouraged to leave EI out of the title of the text to avoid any negative biases about EI.[31] It would be helpful to move past the biases and look at the literature that clearly states that there are positive outcomes when EI is used. Relationships and connections are built through developing positive communication, effectively managing conflicts, and reducing burnout; leading with EI ensures relationship and rapport building, positive communication, effective conflict managment, and a reduction in burnout.

With these things in mind, it would be ideal to embed EI development within medical education but these authors recognize that there is already an overcrowding of the undergraduate and graduate medical education curriculum. Fortunately, EI can be developed or modified at any point, so choosing it as a personal growth goal in practice is a great option. Consider asking for a professional coach who can help and guide with this change.[27]

SUMMARY

Unlike cognitive intelligence or "g," EI is seen as more fluid in terms of ability to improve competencies. Therefore, EI is highlighted as an opportunity for personal development and change. Improving EI positively influences empathy, communication, conflict management, burnout, and leadership. All of which take relationships, rapport, and connection to the next level.

CLINICS CARE POINTS

- Lead with EI for positive team function and outcomes
- Develop EI because it influences affect and job performance
- Enhance empathy for better relationships
- Manage conflict effectively and positively to avoid toxic cultures

DISCLOSURE

Authors neither have commercial or financial conflicts of interests nor were they funded for the study in this article.

REFERENCES

1. Mayer JD, Salovey P, Caruso DR, et al. Measuring emotional intelligence with the MSCEIT V2. 0. Emotion 2003;3(1):97.
2. Andrei F, Smith MM, Surcinelli P, et al. The trait emotional intelligence questionnaire: internal structure, convergent, criterion, and incremental validity in an italian sample. Meas Eval Couns Development 2016;49(1):34–45.
3. Bar-On R. The Bar-On Emotional Quotient Inventory (EQ-i): Rationale, description and summary of psychometric properties. In: Geher G, editor. Measuring emotional intelligence: Common ground and controversy. Nova Science Publishers; 2004. p. 115–45.
4. Goleman D, Boyatzis R. Emotional and social competence inventory (ESCI). The Hay Group; 2007.
5. Arora S, Ashrafian H, Davis R, et al. Emotional intelligence in medicine: a systematic review through the context of the ACGME competencies. Med Educ 2010; 44(8):749–64.
6. Jung JJ, Borkhoff CM, Jüni P, et al. Non-technical skills for surgeons (NOTSS): Critical appraisal of its measurement properties. Am J Surg 2018;216(5):990–7.
7. Taylor C, Farver C, Stoller JK. Perspective: Can emotional intelligence training serve as an alternative approach to teaching professionalism to residents? Acad Med 2011;86(12):1551–4.
8. White B.A.A., Cola P., Boyatzis R.E., et al., Emotionally Intelligent Leadership in Medicine. Front Psychol, Available at: https://www.frontiersin.org/articles/10.3389/fpsyg.2022.999184/full. Accessed August 20, 2022.
9. Nes E, White BAA, Malek AJ, et al. Building communication and conflict management awareness in surgical education. J Surg Education 2022;79(3):745–52.
10. White BAA, Picchioni A, Gentry L, et al. (in production). Closing the Educational Gap in Surgery: Teaching Team Communication and Conflict Management. American Journal of Surgery 2022;224(6):1488–91.
11. White A, Zapata I, Lenz A, et al. Medical students immersed in a hyper-realistic surgical training environment leads to improved measures of emotional resiliency by both hardiness and emotional intelligence evaluation. Front Psychol 2020;11: 569035.
12. Petrides KV, Perazzo MF, Pérez-Díaz PA, et al. Trait Emotional Intelligence in Surgeons. Front Psychol 2022;13:829084.
13. Sharp G, Bourke L, Rickard MJ. Review of emotional intelligence in health care: an introduction to emotional intelligence for surgeons. ANZ J Surg 2020;90(4): 433–40.
14. Wispé L. The distinction between sympathy and empathy: to call forth a concept, a word is needed. J Pers Soc Psychol 1986;50(2):314.
15. Cuff BM, Brown SJ, Taylor L, et al. Empathy: a review of the concept. Emot Rev 2016;8(2):144–53.
16. Hein G, Singer T. I feel how you feel but not always: the empathic brain and its modulation. Curr Opin Neurobiol 2008;18(2):153–8.
17. O'Boyle EH Jr, Humphrey RH, Pollack JM, et al. The relation between emotional intelligence and job performance: A meta-analysis. J Organizational Behav 2011; 32(5):788–818.
18. Fernández-Rodríguez LJ, Bardales-Zuta VH, San-Martín M, et al. Empathy Enhancement Based on a Semiotics Training Program: A Longitudinal Study in Peruvian Medical Students. Front Psychol 2020;11:567663.

19. Tallman K, Janisse T, Frankel RM, et al. Communication practices of physicians with high patient-satisfaction ratings. Permanente J 2007;11(1):19–29.
20. Chou CL, Cooley L. *Communication Rx: transforming healthcare through relationship-centered communication.* McGraw Hill Professional; 2017.
21. Academy of Communication in Healthcare. ACH. (n.d.). Available at: https://achonline.org/. Accessed August 26, 2022.
22. Boyatzis R, McKee A. Resonant leadership. Boston: Harvard Business School Press; 2005.
23. Lopes PN, Nezlek JB, Extremera N, et al. Emotion regulation and the quality of social interaction: Does the ability to evaluate emotional situations and identify effective responses matter? J Personal 2011;79(2):429–67.
24. Greer LL, Saygi O, Aaldering H, et al. Conflict in medical teams: opportunity or danger?: Conflict in medical teams. Med Educ 2012;46(10):935–42.
25. West CP, Dyrbye LN, Shanafelt TD. Physician burnout: contributors, consequences and solutions. J Intern Med 2018;283(6):516–29.
26. Lee YY, Medford AR, Halim AS. Burnout in physicians. J R Coll Physicians Edinb 2015;45(2):104–7.
27. Boyatzis R, Smith ML, Van Oosten E. Helping people change: coaching with compassion for lifelong learning and growth. Harvard Business Press; 2019.
28. White BAA, Bledsoe C, Hendricks R, et al. A leadership education framework addressing relationship management, burnout, and team trust. Baylor Univ Med Cent Proc 2019, April;32(No. 2):298–300. Taylor & Francis.
29. Quinn JF, Perelli S. First and foremost, physicians: the clinical versus leadership identities of physician leaders. J Health Organ Manag 2016;30(4):711–28.
30. Webb AM, Tsipis NE, McClellan TR, et al. A first step toward understanding best practices in leadership training in undergraduate medical education: a systematic review. Acad Med 2014;89(11):1563–70.
31. Quinn JF, White BAA. Cultivating leadership in medicine. Dubuque: Kendall Hunt Publishing Company; 2019.

The Importance of Diversity, Equity, and Inclusion for Effective, Ethical Leadership

Lisa R. Coleman, MD, MPH[a], Erica D. Taylor, MD, MBA[b],*

KEYWORDS

• Diversity • Equity • Inclusion • Ethical leadership

KEY POINTS

• Diversity, equity, and inclusion (DEI) is crucial for the progress of a competitive institution.
• DEI serves to enhance the advancement of all people from all backgrounds, races, perspectives, and cultures.
• DEI increases the productivity, innovation, reputation, and retention of talent.
• The integration and elevation of DEI is complicated by challenges such as resistance to change and unchecked biases.
• There are effective ways leadership can integrate DEI into their institutional culture and succeed.

INTRODUCTION—WHAT IS DIVERSITY, EQUITY, AND INCLUSION?

Take a moment the next time your find yourself in a room with others. Look to your left, then to your right. Who do you see? Do you see people in the room who look like you, share similar ideas, share your gender? Alternatively, do you see an array of backgrounds, ideologies, and identities? If you are experiencing the former and not the latter, you may be missing out on critical benefits and opportunities for achieving optimal leadership. We are at a critical juncture where leaders and teams are recognizing the value of diversifying groups but have yet to understand the true "why" and "how" of achieving inclusivity and belonging in our field. Through understanding of the true meaning of diversity, equity, and inclusion (DEI), its value and phenotype, leaders will be able to harness the power of creating an environment where all people can thrive and contribute.

Diversity, equity, and inclusion are separate terms woven together to provide institutions a roadmap to creating environments and workforces that are effective and

[a] University of Pennsylvania, Penn Medicine, 3400 Spruce Street, Philadelphia, PA 19104, USA;
[b] Duke University School of Medicine, Duke Health, PO Box 1726, Wake Forest, NC 27587, USA
* Corresponding author.
E-mail address: erica.taylor@duke.edu

Clin Sports Med 42 (2023) 269–280
https://doi.org/10.1016/j.csm.2022.11.002
0278-5919/23/© 2022 Elsevier Inc. All rights reserved.

sportsmed.theclinics.com

maintain high-quality talent. The terms are commonly used interchangeably but, to utilize its full effects, it is necessary to understand each term individually in the context of leadership.

Diversity

The term "diversity" is often associated with dimensions of visible difference but its meaning goes much deeper. Derived from a combination of Latin and old French, its root means to "turn aside."[1] Along those lines, diversity challenges leadership to "turn aside" from a homogenous environment of related peoples and ideas and lead their organizations into a world rich with people who differ in race and ethnicity, gender, ideologies, beliefs, learning styles, religions, personalities, abilities, socioeconomics, and several other aspects of individuality. It is important that leaders consider an inclusive context of diversity and unlock its importance. Heterogeneity creates an environment where peoples of different skills and tools can work together to create new innovations and solutions that were otherwise impossible to recognize if only single-tone perspectives were brought to the table.[2] This introduces the relatively newer concept of the "diversity bonus."[2] The "diversity bonus" is a term used to describe the power of bringing together individuals with diverse characteristics and minimal skill overlap in a way that produces better outcomes and new ideas.[2]

There are some organizations who have a set framework of what they subjectively believe makes the best candidates for a team. By using such rigid standards, these organizations do not have the chance to experience diversity bonuses because they filter out any candidate that deviates from their norm.[3] These individuals, even though high quality according to these subjective standards, do not add any diversity bonuses because they bring similar overlapping skills to the group.[2]

Case Example #1: Company "Alpha" has a hiring screen that only allows for candidates with certification test scores of the 90th percentile or higher and requires each applicant to have experience with project funding to be reviewed. By this methodology, it is likely that they will hire candidates with similar backgrounds and skill sets. Through this process, Susan and Michael are hired. They have similar certification scores and experience with project funding. They are given a task to find alternative ways to fund a product design to make the product more affordable while maintaining its effectiveness and marketability. However, although Susan and Michael both have high level scores and experience with funding multiple projects, their ability to create an array of solutions to present to the leadership is a struggle. Because they both have similar overlapping skills and backgrounds, they are creating similar solutions, and not necessarily the best solution. There is no diversity bonus.

Case Example #2: Company Alpha has decided to become active in diversifying their teams and reviews the applications with a broader lens of inclusivity. They find the application of Kenya, whose test scores are slightly below company average, yet she has experience with project funding. On closer review, they see each of the projects she managed was backed by significant stakeholder contributions while maintaining the quality and marketability of the products. Kenya comes from a low socioeconomic background and could not afford the same resources as Susan and Michael. As a result, she possesses an understanding of how to identify and negotiate with stakeholders. In addition, she was excellent at writing and used those skills to compose compelling proposals and obtain further funding resources. By adding Kenya to the team, she offers a new skill set, which will produce diversity bonuses. In this case, the diversity bonus for the team includes composing successful proposals, identifying a broader range of stakeholders, and negotiating significant investments. In addition, Michael and Susan are able to confer test-taking skills to help

Kenya increase her scores, which adds another bonus to the company dynamic. This will further attract more high-quality talent.[4] Hence the power of team diversity.

Equity

Equity is access to resources and opportunities through elimination of obstacles that limit one's ability to achieve success through talent and skills.[5] In other words, equity levels the playing field so that disparities are not a barrier to achieve a goal.[6] Disparities can occur when qualities and attributes privy to discrimination, such as race, gender, and socioeconomic status, put certain populations at a disadvantage irrespective of their innate ability.[6] Equity is not the same as equality. Equality is when everyone gets equal resources.[7] Equity is when everyone gets the resources they need to achieve quality outcomes.[7,8] For example, in **Fig. 1**, you have 3 people of varying heights, each trying to reach for a cup. Each has the skill to grab the cup but each does not have access to the cup based on their height (an attribute that leads to a disparity). With equality, each is given the same height stool. Although they are all given equal amounts of resources, it may not be enough to overcome certain

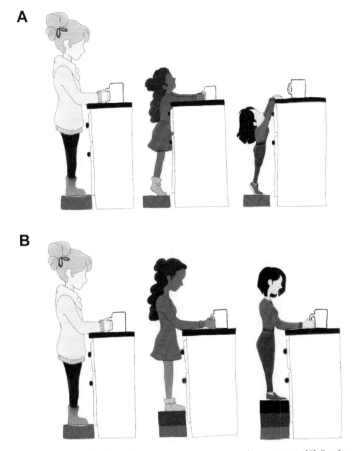

Fig. 1. Equality vs Equity. (*A*) Equality—everyone gets equal resources. (*B*) Equity—access to resources and opportunities to achieve success by eliminating disparities to achieve success.

disparities. However, equity allocates resources so that everyone has access enough to use their arms (skills) to grab the cup (goal).

Of note, it is important to acknowledge the limitation of imagery and definitions of equity because it is easy to assume that the individual needing different resources has personal shortcomings that are a reflection of their innate value. That is certainly not the case. In fact, it is often the system itself that is skewed in a direction that favors one group over another. As a segue from equity, we often hear the term "justice" included in leadership discussions, as an acknowledgement that there are disparities built into system processes that are contributing to these challenges. For leaders, there is a call to address both equity (providing the appropriate resources to an individual to promote their ability to be successful) while also, in parallel, restructuring the processes that may be widening these gaps.

Inclusion

Inclusion involves creating a culture and environment that supports and fosters the talents of individuals through equality fairness, openness, and belonging.[9–11] Inclusion is one of the most important concepts of DEI because it helps to retain the diverse talent that has been recruited and also addresses the desires of belonging that are innate in all humans.[4] It is impossible to reap diversity bonuses if the recruited talent consistently leaves or is dismissed. For example, residency programs across the United States may inadvertently counteract diversity bonuses when an inclusive culture is not also present.[12] Within the disciplines of surgery, this has led to an unprecedented 12% of underrepresented minorities being dismissed from their positions at a higher rate than their White counterparts (2% White residents dismissed).[13] In orthopedic surgery, an article published in 2020 found that Black residents make up almost 6% of orthopedic residents, and more than 17% of them were either dismissed or left the field.[14] Residents report that they were terminated or left due to a lack of an inclusive culture filled with bias, discrimination, intolerance for their diversity contribution, and a lack of opportunities for advancement.[13] The point of diversity is creating an environment of individuals with different experiences, talents, and skills to foster massive success. For that to happen, diverse members of the team need to feel supported, recognized, and validated for their contributions through a culture of respect and belonging.[15] Only then will a team be able to effectively use their full arsenal of skills and abilities to produce diversity bonuses.[3]

Putting it all together, *diversity* is the force that creates an environment where people with different backgrounds, skills, and ideas can come together to contribute to the forward movement of an organization. It provides additive "bonuses" that outpace homogenous environments.[2] *Equity* grants access for diversity to happen. It levels the playing field by acknowledging and overcoming disparate resources so those with qualifying talent can compete in fair competition.[7,8] Finally, *inclusion* allows for the retention of diversity and the bonuses it provides, permitting members of our teams to invest in an environment and make significant contributions, thus strengthening an organization's value.[15]

Misconceptions of Diversity, Equity, and Inclusion

Now that there is a better understanding of how leadership can implement DEI, let us review how misconceptions of DEI by leadership can lead to contradictory results.

DEI is not charity work. According to Jill Davis Kone, the VP and marketing manager of global super diversity at JP Morgan Chase, DEI is a business imperative.[16] The United States is a country that has been rapidly diversifying with more demand coming from minority communities. For an institution to guarantee sustainability and longevity, it is important to foster relationships with these communities. Per Kone, DEI is a business imperative because it causes companies to seek individuals with differing perspectives, approaches, and cultural knowledge that leads to better product development and innovations. So, institutions stagnant in their DEI efforts will begin to fall behind due to inability to connect to the community they are targeting. Organizations, particularly in health care, are recognizing the evolution of DEI effort from optional volunteerism to intentional efforts to decrease morbidity and mortality, thus impacting and saving human lives through health equity. Implementation of the principles of DEI by leadership mandates the restructuring of organizational protocols and processes that are antithetical to achievement of an inclusive environment where all can thrive. This is challenging to do but critical to growth and success of teams.

DEI is not favoring one group of people for another. There has been a misconception that the advancement of one group of people means the demotion of another group of people.[17] For example, this is explained by the term "zero-sum game."[18] According to Norton and Sommers, there have been concerns of "anti-White bias"—better outcomes for Black people will result in worse outcomes for White people, despite the data showing otherwise.[17,18] For example, White households are 13 times more wealthy than Black households with the gap widening despite dedicated programs for minority communities.[19,20] Further, of the practicing orthopedic surgeons, only 1.5% are Black despite increasing access of pipeline programming.[14] DEI is not an "us vs them" approach but rather a unifying force that allows differences between people to be tools that elevate every group of people. DEI does not take away opportunities from a group of people to give another group of people more opportunities. It creates more resources and opens access so everyone can have chances to succeed.

DEI does NOT destroy or underhand traditions. DEI equips traditions to survive the changing times, as demonstrated in the example below.

Case Example #3: Medical School "Beta" has a tradition where a legacy student from physician's families reads the Hippocratic oath at graduation. It is a tradition that has been long-standing since the start of the school. One year, when nominations for this honor were being handed out, it was suggested that the honor include a first-generation student. At first, there was some resistance, especially from the executive level because the change was seen as the destruction of a tradition. In addition, there was fear that certain donors would interpret this change as an honor taken away from their legacy family members. A diverse think-tank of students and faculty was created. This team produced a proposal that explained the importance of the first-generation student. Allowing a first-generation student to share the honor of reading the Hippocratic oath with a legacy student would allow the institution to pay homage to those who started the legacies in the first place. The first-generation doctor experiences unique hardships and breakthroughs that allow for a strong foundation of legacy physician families to be built and maintained. By creating opportunity for a first-generation doctor to share the stage with an established legacy, it allowed for remembrance of contributions within a family while also celebrating new precedents of excellence. Now, at Beta, there is a new tradition of a first generation to represent the beginning of excellence and a legacy to represent the continuance of excellence that read the hypocritic oath at graduation together. DEI adds to tradition and ensures its lasting effect for future generations.

Fostering Diversity, Equity, and Inclusion: a Critical Leadership Tenet

With the understanding of the language and context behind DEI, it is important to recognize these principles as critical leadership tenets for individuals serving in organizational influential roles. Increasing research has studied the effects of DEI on organizations. Commonly reported benefits are increased profitability and production, retaining and attracting talent, increasing innovative capabilities, and elevating reputation.[21]

The Business Case

Profitability/Productivity—A frequent question for many companies, including health-care systems, is how diversity affects business-driven metrics. Several companies have conducted massive global studies and have found promising results. A study done by McKinsey & Company, that included more than 1000 different coanies across 15 countries, found that the most diverse companies had 25% more likely hood to obtain profits above the industry average compared with less diverse companies.[10] Research from Development Dimensions International found that among 2488 companies across different countries, the ones with increased DEI efforts had leaders that were twice as likely to work together, creating solutions that produced 1.5 times more sustained profitable growth.[22] Women in business and management (WBM) found that among 13,000 companies in 70 countries, those that had increased gender diversity experienced 60% higher profitability and productivity.[23]

Innovation—Creating an inclusive environment allows for the creation of a safe space in which diverse talent can work together at their full capacity to produce new and innovating products. Per WBM, companies that were active in creating inclusive cultures saw a 59.1% increase in creativity, innovation, and openness.[23] When groups of differing individuals come together, performance is improved through wider variety of skills and perspectives. In addition, due to these differing perspectives, this can create areas of friction and discourse. Practically, this is desirable for encouragement of deeper deliberation and avoidance of groupthink and conformity.[24] Studies have shown that when individuals are in homogenous groups, there is an increased tendency to rely on other's opinions and decisions. There is an innate bias in trusting the judgement of those who have similar identities, as opposed to those who do not, thus the inclination to conform.[25] Diversity encourages the discourse that leads to robust solutions.[25] This is particularly important in health care when deliberating on diagnosis and best practices. A study found that medical teams of increasing diversity and inclusivity demonstrated an increase in diagnostic accuracy, patient satisfaction, and health care utilization and access. These positive findings were attributed to improvement in doctor–patient communications and relationships.[26]

Reputation—Reputation is a common top priority for health-care organizations and leaders. It represents the perception of an organization's mission, ethics, and ability to deliver results.[27] Reputation can be a determining factor for recruiting high-quality talent, obtaining needed financial stakeholders, and attracting consumers to use services.[27] Implementation of DEI effort is a powerful approach to support enhancing an organization's reputation. Per WBM, companies with active DEI efforts were able to increase their reputations by at least 60%.[23] Customers perceiving organizations as diverse and inclusive were more likely to use their services.[28] In addition, organizations with higher diversity were 37.9% more likely to accurately gauge the interests and demands of their target consumers.[23] Another study found that employees linked an organization's diversity and inclusion efforts to their degree of ethics and virtue.[29] When employees thought that an organization was diverse and inclusive, they saw the company as more ethical and hence reciprocated behaviors that reflected these ethics to fellow coworkers and within their work.[29]

Talent Retention—An inclusive environment leads to diverse talent being able to use their skills to the best of their abilities because they feel safe and valued.[15] Organizations with active DEI efforts have been found to attract and retain their recruited talent

59.7% more than organizations with less-active DEI efforts.[23] When DEI is prevalent in executive or management roles, it was found that these inclusive leaders were able to unlock the potential of their teams. A study at Harvard found that organizations with inclusive leaders had employees that reported as 42% more likely to be more engaged at work and without intentions to leave their jobs within a year.[30]

Although these areas are business-driven outcomes to support embrace of DEI, leaders must also place value, if not higher, on the ethical and moral imperative of creating a culture of respect and belonging for all.

The Fairness Case

Diversity, equity, and inclusion: ethical considerations for leaders

It is no secret that DEI does benefit institutions at the organizational and individual level. For DEI to thrive, ethical considerations must be acknowledged.

Homogeneity—The first ethical consideration brought to light is the unchallenged homogeneity. Across the board, DEI is challenged on every level for its efficacy and ability to profit an organization, yet homogeneity is rarely required to prove itself.[3] Homogeneity or "sameness" is the default of society. It provides a "standard," or something that society can use to determine the value of a person, product, or idea. Often in organizations, the White, male, heterosexual, cis-gender, able-bodied person is the prototype and is rarely asked to prove their value.[3] Homogeneity is convenient and comfortable, which is why conformity exists. It is challenging to combat the convenience homogeneity provides because it does not necessarily rock the boat. Studies have shown people are more likely to trust the judgements of those who look like them leading to requiring less deliberation, which is easier than the challenging engagement of diverse opinions and perspectives that can cause a healthy friction that can produce diversity bonuses.[2,24] However, because of the perceived inconvenience of diversity, it often is discussed as an optional part of leadership value.[3,25]

Policy and Culture—Currently, barriers to DEI are not routinely addressed in policy or culture. According to the theory of the social-ecologic model for behavioral changes, behavior is influenced by multiple levels from the individual to interpersonal, organizational, community, and policies and laws.[31] A change at one level may not produce a behavior change and often requires change at multiple levels. Many institutions have policies such as grievance reporting systems that are, in theory, supposed to identify sources of discrimination and prevent them from propagating further. In reality, these systems are often flawed and can actually support heightened discriminatory and noninclusive behaviors. Investigations have found that many grievance procedures filed with the US Equal Employment Opportunity Commission have led to many cases of retaliation against the people who file complaints.[32,33] In addition to retaliation, there is the issue of the extreme anonymity associated with investigations into discrimination in the workplace. Investigations are commonly carried out without anyone knowing about it.[33] Although intending to protect the identity of the victim, there is also required protection of the accused and makes it harder for a pattern of discrimination and noninclusive behavior to be recognized and reported.[33] This often leaves the victim feeling like the accused is not held accountable, leading to talent leaving the institution.[33] In addition, substantial amounts of evidence are required to prove discrimination and noninclusive behaviors. This takes time, leaving victims to weather the storm in harsh environments for extended time periods.[33] It should also be noted that diverse individuals are often the subject of reporting at a rate higher than those who are part of majority groups when exercising the same behavior.

Values and Unaddressed Bias—Important, DEI requires leadership to honestly evaluate their values and face their own implicit biases. When the word "bias" is mentioned, it is often incorrectly associated with extremes such as racism, sexism, and hatred. However, the bias mentioned here are ones that often go unrecognized, for example, stereotyping. Stereotypes are subjective assumptions used to categorize individuals to quickly understand them.[34,35] One such trouble stereotype is that Black people lack advancement in institutions because they lack work ethic or are lazy.[36] This is commonly seen in training environments when minority residents are perceived as "not up for the job."[12] This can also lead to gaslighting, where diverse residents are scrutinized more severely for mistakes than majority counterparts. This leads to a vicious cycle of closer monitoring, evaluators seeing more mistakes (selection bias), and then an eventual fulfillment of the initial stereotype that diverse residents are not as hardworking or capable as others. In reality, these disparities and lack of fairness in evaluation may result from unchecked biases in leadership.[36,37] Indeed, it is difficult to admit that one may have misjudged a person due to unfounded perceptions of group of people based on attributes that are not objectively true. So, what can leadership do to use DEI to create a culture of respect and belonging in which all can thrive?

How Leadership can Embrace Diversity, Equity, and Inclusion to Make Organizations Competitive and Effective

Recognize That DEI is Challenging—Bringing together a diverse group of people with differing perspectives, skills, and experience can produce friction. It is in these moments of friction that leadership should rely on maintaining a culture of good communication skills such as nonviolent communication (NVC). NVC is a method of communication where a viewpoint is verbally acknowledged by the listener before the listener gives a rebuttal.[38] By acknowledging the speaker's point of view, it allows the speaker to feel valued and heard. This enables the speaker to become an active listener instead of being distracted by thoughts of continuing to make their point. In addition, to good communication, it is also important to recognize that diverse teams will still have failures. Because DEI can be challenging, it is tempting to make easier conclusions that diversity does not work instead of exploring the possibilities of other important pitfalls such as implicit biases, suboptimal leadership teams, and malaigned strategy and inadequate execution.[3]

Be Consistent in Everyday Actions—Celebrating big holidays or having special diversity events are well intended actions to support DEI efforts. However, showing those commitments consistently in everyday activities can be more impactful than intermittent grand gestures.[39] For example, knowing the names of team members and pronouncing them correctly yields significant increases in inclusion.[39] A name is an identity and taking time to consistently do this simple gesture shows inclusive leadership through valuing one's identity and culture. Another small gesture is to take time to understand other background and lived experiences, and find ways to integrate them into the work culture.[39] This can take the form of asking thoughtful questions over coffee, making sure team social events are inclusive, and allowing employees time for wellness.

Seek Feedback—Improvement is made through awareness and collecting data. Leaders should ask for honest feedback from team members about how they are doing as an inclusive leader. By humbly seeking feedback, leadership sets an example that despite their own beliefs, expertise, and experience, their goal is to allow a space for alternative views to be presented.[2] Health care is a dynamic industry, and one has to be flexible, humble, and be willing to learn new things, as well as have a willingness to be wrong.[39]

Promote DEI Properly and Recognize its Value—In many institutions, health-care executive teams are homogenous. A survey from the Center for Talent Innovation found that most men with leadership positions reported that they did not have time to be involved in DEI efforts. This points to an unfortunate reality that institutions still perceive DEI as "optional" instead of essential to their success. A way to reverse this is to promote DEI in a way that helps leaders to see that these values are contributing to their goals, instead of taking time away from achieving them.[4,40] This can be presented as incentives to inclusive practices, such as more weight given to creating an inclusive culture on performance reviews, linking value to the recruitment and retention of diverse talent, and presenting current data of the benefit of more diverse teams, which can increase motivation to be part of the change.[40]

Leadership Development Programs—DEI efforts among leadership may be stagnant due to knowledge gaps surrounding of how to be an inclusive leader. As a part of DEI efforts, institutions should include leadership development as an integral part of creating an inclusive culture.[40] There are several resources and groups available to help facilitate availability of these opportunities. For example, the Orthopaedic Diversity Leadership Consortium (ODLC) serves as a network of orthopedic diversity leaders whose mission is to optimize the effectiveness and sustainability of diversity efforts by sharing best practices and innovative strategies for success.[41] Organizations such as ODLC have provided resources for developing DEI leadership skills, including workshops, coaching services, and online certificate classes linked to prominent institutions. Instruction on the pearls of effective leadership domains, combined with an understanding of the fundamentals of DEI, has produced a very powerful set of skills for leaders to drive organizational change.

In conclusion, DEI is a powerful tool and each of its components is of great value to the advancement of an institution, especially in health care. With the increasing diversity of our population—humans in need of equitable health care, fair and just work environments, and inclusive learning experiences—DEI becomes a business and fairness imperative. It is critical for health-care leaders to recruit and nurture the diverse talent needed to produce the organizational while building and maintaining important relationships within the communities we all serve.

CLINICS CARE POINTS

- DEI increases a team's performance through heterogenous input of differing ideas and perspectives, leading to positive outcomes of increased diagnostic accuracy, patient satisfaction, and quality of care.

- DEI can be difficult to establish due to the presence of unaddressed biases and ineffective policies against discrimination and noninclusive behaviors.

- Intentional valuation of DEI efforts through inclusive leadership curriculums and metrics can help leaders recognize DEI as a critical asset to organizational success and the equitable care of humans.

DISCLOSURE

L.R. Coleman has no disclosures. E.D. Taylor: Zimmer Biomet: Faculty Research Grant. DePuy Synthes: Consultant. Stryker: Consultant.

REFERENCES

1. Diversity, n. In: Oxford English Dictionary. June 2022. Available at: https://www-oed-com.proxy.library.upenn.edu/view/Entry/56064?redirectedFrom=diversity. Accessed July 30, 2022.
2. Paige SE. Diversity bonuses: the idea. In: Lewis E, Cantor N, editors. The diversity bonus: how great teams pay off in the knowledge economy. Princton, NJ: Princeton University Press; 2017. p. 13–52.
3. Phillips KW, Paige SE. What is the real value of diversity in organizations? Questioning our assumptions. In: Lewis E, Cantor N, editors. The diversity bonus: how great teams pay off in the knowledge economy. Princton, NJ: Princeton University Press; 2017. p. 13–52.
4. Heskett J. Why Don't More Organizations Understand the Power of Diversity and Inclusion? Harv Business Sch Working Knowledge, Business Res Business Leaders. 2020. Available at: https://hbswk.hbs.edu/item/why-don-t-more-organizations-understand-the-power-of-diversity-and-inclusion. Accessed July 30, 2022.
5. U.S. Department of Health and Human Services. Paving the Road to Health Equity. Centers for Disease Control and Prevention. 2020. Available at: https://www.cdc.gov/minorityhealth/publications/health_equity/index.html#:~:text=As%20defined%20by%20the%20U.S.,outcomes%20than%20individual%2Dlevel%20factors. Accessed July 20, 2022.
6. Braveman P. What are health disparities and health equity? We need to be clear. Public Health Rep 2014;129(Suppl 2):5–8.
7. Braveman P, Gruskin S. Defining equity in health. J Epidemial Community Health 2003;57(4):254–8.
8. International Conference on Primary Health Care. Declaration Alma-ata *WHO Chron* 1978;32(11):428–30.
9. U.S. Department of Housing and Urban Development. Diversity and Inclusion Definitions. U.S. Department of Housing and Urban Development. Available at: https://www.hud.gov/program_offices/administration/admabout/diversity_inclusion/definitions. Accessed July 20, 2022.
10. Dixon-Fyle S, Hunt V, Dolan K, et al. Diversity wins: how inclusion matters. McKinsey & Company; 2020.
11. Rosenkranz KM, Arora TK, Termuhlen PM, et al. Diversity, Equity and Inclusion in Medicine: Why It Matters and How do We Achieve It? J Surg Educ 2021;78(4):1058–65.
12. McFarling UL. 'It was stolen from me': Black doctors are forced out of training programs at far higher rates than white residents. STAT. 2022. Available at: https://www.statnews.com/2022/06/20/black-doctors-forced-out-of-training-programs-at-far-higher-rates-than-white-residents/. Accessed July 30, 2022.
13. McDade W. Diversity and Inclusion in Graduate Medical Education. Accreditation Council for Graduate Medical Education. 2019. Available at: https://southernhospitalmedicine.org/wp-content/uploads/2019/10/McDade-ACGME-SHM-Presentation-McDade-Final.pdf. Accessed July 30, 2022.
14. McDonald TC, Drake LC, Replogle WH, et al. Barriers to Increasing Diversity in Orthopaedics: The Residency Program Perspective. JB JS Open Access 2020; 5(2):e0007.
15. Paige SE. Practice: D&T + D&I. In: Lewis E, Cantor N, editors. The diversity bonus: how great teams pay off in the knowledge economy. Princton, NJ: Princeton University Press; 2017. p. 209–23.

16. Kone JD. 2. S02:E02 – Supplier Diversity is Not a Handout with Jill Davis Kone. Supplier Diversity TV. October 15-16, 2018. Available at: https://youtu.be/PnC_PkJ_EK0. Accessed August 6, 2022.

17. McGhee H. The sum of us: what racism costs everyone and how we can prosper together. Manhattan, NY: Random House Publishing Group; 2021.

18. Norton MI, Sommers SR. Whites see racism as a zero-sum game that they are now losing. Perspect Psychol Sci 2011;6(3):215–8.

19. McIntosh K, Moss E, Nunn R, et al. Examining the Black-white wealth gap. Brookings 2020. Available at: https://www.brookings.edu/blog/up-front/2020/02/27/examining-the-black-white-wealth-gap/. Accessed July 30, 2022.

20. Brown A, Atske S. Black Americans have made gains in U.S. political leadership, but gaps remain. Pew Res Cent 2021. Available at: https://www.pewresearch.org/fact-tank/2021/01/22/black-americans-have-made-gains-in-u-s-political-leadership-but-gaps-remain/. Accessed July 30, 2022.

21. Catalyst. Quick Take: Why Diversity and Inclusion Matter. Catalyst Inc. June 24. 2020. Available at: https://www.catalyst.org/research/why-diversity-and-inclusion-matter/. Accessed August 6, 2022.

22. Sinar E, Wellins RS, Canwell AL, et al. Global leadership forecast 2018: 25 research insights to fuel your people strategy: ASEAN, 2018, Development Dimensions International, Inc, The Conference Board Inc, EYGM limited.

23. Chang JH, Viveros JL, Wirth L. Women in Business and Management: the business case for change. 2nd edition. Geneva: International Labour Organization; 2019.

24. Gomez LE, Bernet P. Diversity improves performance and outcomes. J Natl Med Assoc 2019;111(4):383–92.

25. Gaither SE, Apfelbaum EP, Birnbaum HJ, et al. Mere membership in racially diverse groups reduces conformity. Social Psychologic Personal Sci 2018;9(4):402–10.

26. LaVeist TA, Nuru-Jeter A, Jones KE. The association of doctor-patient race concordance with health services utilization. J Public Health Policy 2003;24(3–4):312–23.

27. Gibson D, Gonzales JL, Castanon J. The importance of reputation and the role of public relations. Public Relations Q 2006;51(3):15.

28. Zalis S. Inclusive ads are affecting consumer behavior, according to new research. The Female Quotient, Google/Ipsos. 2019. Available at: https://www.thinkwithgoogle.com/future-of-marketing/management-and-culture/diversity-and-inclusion/thought-leadership-marketing-diversity-inclusion/. Accessed August 6, 2022.

29. Rabl T, Triana MDC, Byun SY, et al. Diversity Management Efforts as an Ethical Responsibility: How Employees' Perceptions of an Organizational Integration and Learning Approach to Diversity Affect Employee Behavior. J Business Ethics 2020;161:531–50.

30. Sherbin L, Rashid R. Diversity doesn't stick without inclusion. Harvard business review. Cambridge, MA: Harvard Business School Publishing Corporation; 2017. p. 1–5.

31. National Cancer Institute. Part 2: theories and applications. Bethesda, MD: U.S. Department of Health and Human Services, National Institutes of Health; 2005. p. 9–35.

32. U.S. Equal Employment Opportunity Commission. Retaliation-Based Charges (Charges filed with EEOC) FY 1997 – FY 2021. Available at: https://www.eeoc.

gov/statistics/retaliation-based-charges-charges-filed-eeoc-fy-1997-fy-2021. Accessed August 6, 2022.

33. Dobbin F, Kalev A. Making discrimination and harassment compliant systems better. 1st edition. What works? Evidence-based ideas to increase diversity, equity, and inclusion in the workplace. Amherst, MA: University of Massachusetts Amherst; 2018. p. 24–30.

34. Quinn K, Macrae C, Bodenhausen G. Stereotyping and impression formation: how categorical thinking shapes person perception. In: Hogg MA, Cooper J, editors. The SAGE handbook of social psychology: concise student edition. SAGE Publications Ltd; 2007. p. 68–92. https://doi.org/10.4135/9781848608221.n4.

35. Berrey E, Nelson RL, Neilsen LB. Stereotyping and the reinscription of race, sex, disability, and age heirarchies. Rights on trial: how workplace discrimination law perpetuates inequality. Chicago, IL: University of Chicago Press; 2017. p. 225–59.

36. Sears DO, Henry PJ. The origins of symbolic racism. J Pers Soc Psychol 2003; 85(2):259–75.

37. Bielby WT. Minimizing workplace gender and racial bias. Contemp Sociol 2000; 29(1):120–9.

38. Rosenberg MB, Chopra D. Nonviolent communication: a language of life: life-changing tools for healthy relationships. Encinitas, CA: PuddleDancer Press; 2015.

39. Bourke J, Titus A. Why Inclusive Leaders are Good for Organizations, and How to Become One. Harv Business 2019. Available at: https://hbr.org/2019/03/why-inclusive-leaders-are-good-for-organizations-and-how-to-become-one. Accessed August 10, 2022.

40. Newman EA, Waljee J, Dimick JB, et al. Eliminating Institutional Barriers to Career Advancement for Diverse Faculty in Academic Surgery. Ann Surg 2019; 270(1):23–5.

41. Orthopaedic Diversity Leadership Consortium. Our Mission. ODLC. 2022. Available at: https://orthodiversity.org/about-odlc/mission/. Accessed August 10, 2022.

Putting it all together/Lessons from Outside

Insights on Coaching, Mentorship, and Leadership from Business to Health Care

Sanyin Siang, MBA

KEYWORDS

- Coaching • Mentorship • Leadership • Health care • Power dynamic • Pandemic
- Aspirations • Expectations

KEY POINTS

- The coronavirus disease 2019 pandemic accelerated many global trends, including how we work, how we lead, and how we interact with each other.
- There has been a power shift in the power dynamic that once drove institutions to an infrastructure and operating framework that encourages new employee expectations, including the humanization of leadership from those in power.
- The health-care sector must match its technical competence with new standards of leadership, including leader-as-coach and leader-as-mentor.

SIX INSIGHTS WE CAN BRING FROM THE CORPORATE WORLD CAN BENEFIT THE HEALTH-CARE EXPERIENCE

1. Everyone wants to be seen. From orderlies to patients, surgeons to interns, department heads to volunteers—they all want leadership notice, respect, and recognition.
2. Everyone wants to be heard. Workers will seek someone who hears them as surely as water seeks its own level. Active listening remains a good tactic but employees also look for honesty and authenticity.
3. Everyone needs recognition. Health-care leaders must recognize and respect the individual employee's contribution. However, leaders must frame that recognition to accentuate that individual's interdependence with the whole.
4. Everyone has expectations and aspirations. People gravitate to those who espouse, affirm, and execute shared values and aspirations. Leaders of consequence model the authentic and ethical qualities that enable and empower worker potential.

Fuqua/Coach K Center on Leadership & Ethics, Fuqua School of Business, Box 90120, 100 Fuqua Drive, Durham, NC 27708, USA
E-mail address: Sanyin.siang@duke.edu

Clin Sports Med 42 (2023) 281–289
https://doi.org/10.1016/j.csm.2022.12.001
0278-5919/23/© 2022 Elsevier Inc. All rights reserved.

5. Everyone wants connection. A dynamism arises from our interaction with others. Moreover, this may be truer for those in health care where people want to pursue a purpose higher than themselves.
6. Everyone seeks a leader. Teams of consequence follow leaders who know and care for them. This power does not come with title, authority, or project management. Leadership originates from a human-to-human ecosystem where leaders model and inspire collaborative behaviors.

In my work as an executive coach, educator, and head of a premier leadership center at Duke University, I have had a unique horizontal vantage point. I work with CEOs, board directors, and entrepreneurs, across public, private, and social sectors. The diversity of these relationships gives me an inside look into patterns of leadership. While on the surface, the chair of the Joint Chiefs of Staff, the CEO of a startup who is transforming robotics, or a Nobel Laureate who runs a research laboratory may seem to lead very different organizations, the levers they pull to lead effectively are surprisingly similar. Among nuanced differences, we can draw analogies for leading between the corporate world, the science bench—and even health care.

One consistency that every context must deal with is a changing environment. Moreover, this changing environment has made it so the leadership playbook used by our predecessors is not as easily applicable. Here are some of the key changes.

First, the coronavirus disease 2019 (COVID-19) pandemic accelerated many global trends, including how we work, how we lead, and how we interact with one another. Moreover, while the crisis seems to have plateaued, we have yet to come to terms with its effects. From mom-and-pop businesses to global enterprises, organizations and their leaders struggled to cope, adapt, and survive.

Second, there has also been a shift in the power dynamics that once drove institutions and individuals. Previously, legacy employers have told employees, "You can stay with us as long as you want to be with us (or as long as we need you)." However, organizations have deployed work to remote situations. Government subsidies have allowed people to reassess their purpose. The Millennials and Z Generation have come of age. Moreover, a talent shortage amid The Great Resignation has tested anxious recruiters everywhere.

We now see employees staying with companies at will. Workers have new expectations, including the humanization of leadership from those in positions of power. They seek work with companies that treat employees as well as their customers. Moreover, talent wants an infrastructure and operating framework that encourages and empowers interdependencies.

Some pundits promised a "new normal." They predicted "a brave new world" would arise after the pandemic. In fact, we can say that ours is no longer a linear world. Now, the health-care universe presents unique and complex challenges. Its protocols and personalities create a power dynamic that often stretches health care's mission "to do no harm."

I want to surface some of the insights that I have seen in the corporate world around leadership, coaching, and mentoring for consideration in the health-care sector. Just as technical competencies in the business world—competencies such as strategy, marketing, or finance—all need to be supplemented and contextualized in good, sturdy leadership, the health-care sector must match its technical competencies with new standards of leadership. These new standards include the leader-as-coach and the leader-as-mentor. Whether one is a first-year resident, a senior nurse, or a seasoned physician attending, there is a responsibility to be a leader-coach, a leader-mentor to help raise the standards of excellence for the team and patient care. Health-care workers are uniquely positioned to change the industry's power dynamic.

The Current Context

Surveys by Newsweek,[1] YouGov.com,[2] Gallup,[3] and others show a decline in patient confidence and satisfaction. This broad and deep dissatisfaction coincides with other foundational shifts in relationships between institutions and individuals. People feel a new freedom to confront and reject legacy organizations they find paralyzed by age and misaligned purpose. They quit their careers quietly as organizations decline into static maintenance.

The US Bureau of Labor Statistics[4] notes that September 2022 saw health care add 60,000 and has returned to its February 2020 level. Still, Morning Consult[5] parses this in more detail:

- "18% of health care workers have quit their jobs during the COVID-19 pandemic, while another 12% have been laid off.
- Among health care workers who have kept their jobs during the pandemic, 31% have considered leaving.
- 79% of health care professionals said the national worker shortage has affected them and their place of work."

Signs indicate some plateauing, yet the pandemic experience has left health-care personnel deeply affected physically and emotionally. Ed Yong writes for The Atlantic,[6] "Healthcare workers aren't quitting because they can't handle their jobs. They're quitting because they can't handle being unable to do their jobs."

COVID incarceration, remote work, government subsidies, and more have contributed to "The Great Resignation." However, under the debate on its origin, this sea change reveals that employees have new expectations, more significant uncertainty, and a desire for interdependencies. In this complex environment, it is no longer about the individual contributor but the *team*. Amid the unprecedented emotional traumas in pandemic health care, people have learned they are the most potent assets in an organization—not the technology. People will prosper in an environment that empowers a confident expectation of humanized leadership from those in power.

Organizations have the opportunity to shift from a traditional hierarchy toward a better employee experience. Moreover, I think this shift to a different power dynamic means adopting the coaching, mentoring, and leading behaviors that have made such a powerful impact on contemporary business organizations.

Reimagined Definitions

Employees and customers want an authentic, collaborative experience. However, let me first cite working definitions to differentiate coaching, mentoring, and leading.

- Coaching: People usually think of coaching as the advice and motivation that directs teams to achieve their goals. In addressing individuals, coaching creates an environment where each teammate feels confident in decision-making, leading to change.

My long friendship with Duke's legendary Mike Krzyzewski favors an understanding that great coaching unlocks a person's potential.

We do not expect coaches to hold a player's hand when we watch our favorite sport. Coaches remain on the sidelines except for the occasional time-out to quickly motivate the players.

Good coaches have done their work before teams set foot on the field, court, or pitch. They have drawn a playbook and assigned individual talents to their respective roles. Coaches run drills with players to make motion and tactics part of their muscle memory.

Similarly, the health care's leaders in their role as leader-coaches must draw a picture of the organization's vision and mission. Then, they must select the individual talents with achievement potential. Beyond that, coaches rehearse protocols, tweak skills, and advise on the action at decisive moments.

- Mentoring: ATD[7] (Association for Talent Development) defines "mentoring" as "a reciprocal and collaborative at-will relationship." I like the emphasis on a "collaborative at-will relationship." However, I would add that these relationships ought to build trust. Because each person brings value to the mentoring bond, we must pursue connections with diverse talents.

Young people, especially those in underserved communities, want models with whom they can identify. Health care has no obligation to please them. However, encouraging and sustaining mentoring has significant benefits.

Mentors have work and life experience that values stories. They are wired to tell stories about the organization, its history, and its promise. Mentors love to talk, so health-care organizations should place them with those who love to listen and those who need to know.

In telling stories, mentors communicate their feelings. They make it okay to sympathize and empathize. They use their permission to share to inspire and motivate others.

- Leading: Rather than defining leadership as expertise or positional power, I am drawing on the definition we use at the Fuqua/Coach K Center on Leadership & Ethics—that of leadership as the ability to directly influence the outcome of a goal.

To that end, leaders create a climate of psychological safety. They inspire with consistent behaviors that model how to achieve the promised aspirations. Once established, that culture allows teams and individuals to collaborate, taking actions and making decisions aligned with an organization's goals and core values.

People do lead from the front and from behind. However, they can lead from the middle, too. Leaders become a source of trust in respecting others for their honesty, enthusiasm, and confidence in the future.

Leaders of consequence inspire people to trust in the organization's choice of goals and core values. People want leaders to demonstrate compliance with the organization's values. They want to join the leader on that journey but they also expect the leader to provide the resources for success and remove the necessary barriers to achievement.

Complex hierarchies in organizations can make it challenging to identify leaders. However, organizational charts do not make leaders. Leaders will arise from anywhere if they are passionate about communicating, seeing projects and protocols through, and respecting the staff who make things happen.

Bringing These Insights to Health Care

In our Six Domains of Leadership,[8] my colleagues E. Allen Lind and Sim B. Sitkin, show how "to create a sense of loyalty, trust, community, high aspirations, independent judgment and stewardship" among leader–follower relationships. We think, "In learning about and reflecting on one's own behaviors, in engaging others, and in being open about their perceptions of those behaviors in the context of these 6 domains [of leadership], one can learn to be a better and more effective leader."

We can change, scale, and strengthen health-care operations by adopting insights powerfully effective in business:

Insight #1: everyone wants to be seen
Ask yourself, "What do medical professionals and institutions do to notice the unnoticed?" Everyone wants to be seen. That includes everyone from orderlies to patients, surgeons to interns, department heads to volunteers.

If we watch what happens in everyday settings, we've probably seen those in leadership positions ignore the people serving their lunch in the hospital cafeteria. Caught up with everyday to-do lists, a healthcare provider may fail to welcome or acknowledge a patient's visiting family.

It takes such little effort to recognize the people cleaning up after surgery, the medical admissions clerk at the front desk, or the security guard on duty. They deserve a pat on the back, a tip of the hat, or a simple, sincere smile.

Senior health-care professionals have trained to observe. Residents have trained to shadow. However, these traditions lack engagement. You must bring recognition and acknowledgment to every relationship.

Zulu people use "sawubona" as a greeting such as "hello." However, more literally it means, "I see you." It indexes our ability to see others and help them truly see each other. It affirms that we understand their hopes and goals, appreciate what matters to them, and respect the best version of their fullest selves.

Insight #2: everyone wants to be heard
People have voices, some stronger or louder than others. Before you dismiss those voices as bothersome and irrelevant, understand that workers will seek out someone to hear them as surely as water seeks its own level.

You can stop or redirect that flow with behavior that shows your respect for their remarks. Active listening behaviors—eye contact, nodding, reiterating the employee's words—help. However, workers also look for honesty and authenticity. They will accept a refusal if you explain your position clearly. They will take coaching toward a different goal. Moreover, they will rejoice if you consider their input.

Deep listening remains critical when hearing from culturally diverse or traditionally underserved communities. Their voices come from unique experiences to suggest a different angle on design or deliverables. Writing for the Journal of the National Medical Association,[9] Dr Fatima Stanford noted, "It is important to have a health-care workforce which represents the tapestry of our communities as it relates to race/ethnicity, gender, sexual orientation, immigration status, physical disability status, and socioeconomic level to render the best possible care to our diverse patient populations."

However, this view risks reducing diversity to a numbers game. Health-care professionals should listen for utility and purpose among the numbered voices. Often it just makes good sense to engage with marginalized colleagues because they have a unique voice that better serves the situation or patient.

Insight #3: everyone needs recognition
People follow leaders. Health-care systems assign interns, residents, nurses, and others to "leaders." Institutions put health-care workers into boxes with vertical and horizontal relationships.

These same institutions can fail to respect the new dynamic where the agency for intended outcomes belongs to individuals. Leaders of consequence have risen from the world of command and demand. They recognize that each strategy, plan, and tactic is a system of systems.

Health-care leaders must recognize and respect the individual employee's contribution. However, leaders must frame that recognition to accentuate that individual's interdependence with the whole. Such leaders will create a psychologically safe environment where individuals have the resources and space to develop relationships with their functions, tools, and colleagues. It is best to recognize their unique talent and contribution in the context of the other systems on which they depend or interact.

Insight #4: everyone has expectations and aspirations

People dream. High expectations and ideals drive the health-care workforce. Health-care workers dream of results beyond the minimalist "do no harm." They study, train, and practice to improve the lives of others. Although COVID-19 sorely tested that commitment, pursuing a purpose greater than ourselves sustains the outcomes.

Working people first look to those named to lead. They seek transformational leaders, those who inspire and motivate. People gravitate to those who espouse, affirm, and execute shared values and aspirations. Moreover, leaders of consequence model the authentic and ethical qualities that enable and empower worker potential.

Values cascade down. In health care, the workforce best actualizes the organization's goals when coached, mentored, and led by professionals of character. Leaders who transfer values transform the outcomes of others.

Mary Kay Copeland (International Journal of Leadership Studies[10]) holds that through these transformational leaders, "the goals of the organization become ethical, moral, not self-serving, and focused on the well-being of the followers and organization as a whole. Authentic, ethical, transformational leadership provides an enthusiasm and support for that that is good and moral, and fosters trust and enthusiasm."

In my opinion, workers will not trust leaders who fail to support their objectives. That means knowing what they need. You cannot expect people to give you backing if you do not help them understand what support you need.

- You cannot exercise support *passively*. Giving support does not always mean going along with the aspirations of others. For example, a teammate may be about to make a big mistake. Coaching lets you say, "Do not do that. That is going to be a disaster. Here's why." Mentoring helps you say, "You may not be ready for that just now but here are the gaps I can help you with when you are ready."

Giving support means giving positive strokes, tough love, and constructive feedback.

- You must have the courage to ask for feedback—and to accept and act on it. It may seem counterintuitive but you grow through bad news. You lead with consequence when you tell people they can deliver unwelcome news without repercussion. Their information expands your understanding of the context and consequences. The feedback reveals their capabilities and potential.

Insight #5: everyone wants connection

Humans seek social interaction instinctively. Families, friendships, and fraternities testify to the pull of socialization. A dynamism arises from our interaction with others. Moreover, this may be truer for those in health care where people want to pursue a purpose higher than themselves.

Medical disciplines, departments, and teams hope to succeed in practical and valuable ways. However, they excel when the individual members feel a sense of emotional connectedness. This connection among workers begins with integrating your personal self-awareness with understanding each other and seeing each other as people—with strengths, weaknesses, wisdom, and needs.

Emotional connectedness seems in teams where the members rely on each other. This leaning on and in marks a shared sense of dependency, an interdependency in which each person brings something that helps the entire collective. This interdependency builds the trust of necessity. Teams are not a collection of players. Teams of consequence discover confidence in members' relationships and their joint commitment to achieve a goal.

Of course, you do not always get the teammates you want. As a leader, you must think that your team members are enough. A leader will help everyone think they can hit their target. The challenge requires leaders to grasp the fuller range of value beyond the current expectations. Leaders of consequence envision achievements that stretch the established goals.

Team members bring unique talents and specialized skills to the group. The team's goals require such capabilities. However, the leader must discover and unlock the teammates' respective superpowers. Leaders of consequence coach teams with members with a natural talent for fostering interteam and intrateam relationships. These teammates provide the emotional glue for the team. They cross-pollinate valuable information. Moreover, they increase the joy of work for everyone. It occurs to me that we do record *assists* in sports but we must do the same for workplace teams.

People want a sense of belonging. They seek and thrive in environments that welcome, nurture, and inspire them. They pursue life in a family—worship, sports, military, and more. Such groupings ensure safety, trust, and purpose. Moreover, the members' interdependence, reciprocal respect, and integrated superpowers make things happen.

Insight #6: everybody seeks a leader
People search for guidance. They appreciate those who can make tough decisions. However, leadership does not attach to institution, title, or technical expertise. You may have impressive credentials in finance, marketing, or even management but not have what it takes to lead.

Among all the definitions of "leadership," I find leadership consists of exercising direct influence over others. Leaders of consequence can be challenging but they help team members understand that active decisions serve their best interests. Expertise and experience only matter if people will listen to you and if you can achieve the goals that they want to achieve.

To lead, you must understand attributes do not make a leader. It is about behaviors. The critical behavior lies in the ability to ask questions. You want to ask yourself what you can do to make things happen. You need to know what your team needs to increase its effectiveness. Moreover, it would be best if you asked what you and your team must do to make the organization succeed.

Teams of consequence follow leaders who know and care for them. This power does not come with title, authority, or project management. Leadership rises from a human-to-human ecosystem. Leaders model and inspire collaborative behaviors. They listen and process feedback. They ensure the necessary resources and remove barriers. Then they step out of the way, granting stewardship to those who want to improve things. Leaders of consequence encourage and empower stewardship and agency.

SUMMARY

You Can Change Your Health Care World by Asking a Simple Question of Everyone You Meet Each Day: "How Do You Feel Today?"

The health-care ecosystem has a sense of unique stewardship owed to society. The mission and vision to bring value and improve care to the community attract promising talents to the field. Those who join with romantic aspirations soon find exertion and fatigue in the work. However, this is where leaders come in. Leaders ought to step forward to renew those aspirations, show others the way, and get things done.

I try not to rely too heavily on sport analogies but in this case, it is apt. If you are in a softball game with fellow health-care workers, you know that winning the game requires that you hit, throw, and catch without regard to the rank of others. We need to capture this sense of interplay and hone it in the workplace. We can still respect the roles assigned by medical practice and protocols but play the game with a stronger sense of our places in the team organism.

Health care offers complex challenges. Its noble purpose often brings out the best in the talent it attracts. That same talent leads best when it takes stock of itself. Would-be leaders must take a deep personal inventory of their strengths. They can best display these strengths through a robust, optimistic, and confident coaching, mentoring, and leading strategy.

As coaches, they create a playbook that their teammates can use for playmaking, collaboration, and improvisation. As mentors, they share their stories and experiences but they also listen and learn from the stories told by others. Moreover, as leaders they find and develop talents capable of surpassing current goals and laying out a future for the team.

DISCLOSURE

The author has nothing to disclose.

REFERENCES

1. World's Best Hospitals 2020. 2022. Retrieved from Newsweek: https://www.newsweek.com/best-hospitals-2020/united-states.
2. The Most Popular Hospitals. 2022.). (n.d.). Retrieved from YouGovAmerica: https://today.yougov.com/ratings/health/popularity/hospitals/all.
3. The most popular hospitals. (n.d.). Retrieved from YouGovAmerica: https://today.yougov.com/ratings/health/popularity/hospitals/all.
4. Bureau of Labor Statistics News Release. The employment situation - september 2022. Washington, D.C.: U.S. Department of Labor; 2022. Retrieved from. https://www.bls.gov/news.release/pdf/empsit.pdf.
5. Gooch K. 18% of healthcare workers have quit jobs during pandemic: Morning Consult. 2021. Retrieved from Becker's Hospital Review: https://www.beckershospitalreview.com/workforce/18-of-healthcare-workers-have-quit-jobs-during-pandemic-morning-consult.html.
6. Yong E. Why Health-Care Workers are Quiting in Droves. 2021. Retrieved from The Atlantic: https://www.theatlantic.com/health/archive/2021/11/the-mass-exodus-of-americas-health-care-workers/620713/.
7. What is Mentoring (n.d.). Retrieved from ATD - Association for Training Development: https://www.td.org/talent-development-glossary-terms/what-is-mentoring#:~:text=Mentoring%20is%20a%20reciprocal%20and%20collaborative%20at-will

%20relationship,of%20the%20mentee%E2%80%99s%20growth%2C%20learning%2C%20and%20career%20development.

8. Sitkin S, Lind A. The Six Domains of Leadership. 2008. http://deltaleadership.com/wp-content/uploads/2017/05/Six-Domains-paperwhitepaper-11-.pdf.

9. Stanford F. The Importance of Diversity and Inclusion in the Healthcare Workforce. J Am Med Assoc 2020, June;247–9. Retrieved from. https://www.sciencedirect.com/science/article/abs/pii/S0027968420300663?via%3Dihub.

10. Copeland M. The Emerging Significance of Values Based Leadership: A Literature Review. Int J Leaderships Stud 2014;8(2):105–35. Retrieved from. https://fisherpub.sjf.edu/cgi/viewcontent.cgi?article=1004&context=business_facpub&httpsredir=1&referer=.

Coaching, Mentorship, and Leadership Lessons Learned from Professional Football

James M. Whalen, MSEd, ATC[a], Daryl J. Nelson, MS, LAT, ATC[a],
Ryan J. Whalen, BS, CSCS[b],
Matthew T. Provencher, MD, MBA, MC[b,c],*

KEYWORDS

- Leadership • Mentorship • Coaching • Professional football
- National football league • NFL

KEY POINTS

- Leadership at every level of an organization is paramount to the success of a proffesional football team.
- The most efffective leaders have the ability to mentor those around them and make them great people on and off the field, which stems into successful careers of their own.
- Medical team leadership can take the lessons learned from coaching, leadership, mentorship from professional football and translate that to their own medical team to form a trustowrthy and cohesive ggroup.

INTRODUCTION

Leadership is one of the most covered topics in modern literature and is defined as the ability of an individual or a group of individuals to influence and guide followers or other members of an organization.[1] Nowhere is leadership more visible than on the gridiron. The principles of leadership are apparent in football, from youth leagues, high school, to collegiate, and then especially on Sundays during professional football games when the coach as well as other leaders on the team are asked to lead their team to victory. What the public sees for 3 hours on a Sunday professional football contest is the culmination of a whole offseason, training camp, and an intense week of preparation.

There have been some incredible leaders as coaches, players, and also general management, and ownership in the National Football League. A common thread

[a] New England Patriots, 1 Patriot Place, Foxboro, MA 02035, USA; [b] Steadman Philippon Research Institute, 181 West Meadow Drive Suite 400, Vail, CO 81657, USA; [c] The Steadman Clinic, 181 West Meadow Drive Suite 400, Vail, CO 81657, USA
* Corresponding author. The Steadman Clinic, 181 West Meadow Drive Suite 400, Vail 81657, CO.
E-mail address: mprovencher@thesteadmanclinic.com

Clin Sports Med 42 (2023) 291–299
https://doi.org/10.1016/j.csm.2022.11.009
0278-5919/23/© 2022 Elsevier Inc. All rights reserved.

sportsmed.theclinics.com

between all of these great leaders on the gridiron is that they all followed the philosophy of the ancient philosopher Sun Tzu—"Every Battle is Won Before it is Fought." [2] Football is the ultimate team sport, it is a synchronous combination of skill and strategy. Successful organizations all have a common thread: a management structure that clearly outlines the roadmap for success. Championship organizations are built on creating a successful culture. This starts with ownership providing the support and resources. Vince Lombardi had "The Rules," the 49ers had the "Standards of Performance," and the Patriots have "The Patriot Way." All of these represent basic tenets of leadership to execute the vision of winning on the field.

As leaders carve out their legacy, their impact is not only defined by their victories, but their ability to mentor and develop individuals to lead their own successful programs and organizations. Just as Socrates mentored Plato, we recognize the influence and expansive impact intentional mentorship can have in areas such as sports and medicine. In the sports world, the best example of mentorship are coaching trees. Like a family tree, a coaching tree is a chart that depicts the connections of coaches that have branched out to lead their respective organizations and the main branches from which they came.[3] Coaching trees can reflect not only the direct influence a coach has had on an assistant or intern, but also the adopted philosophic strategies, concepts, and leadership styles drawn from observation.

Professional football has been played for more than 100 years. During this period of time, there are several leadership dynasties that truly stand out: the Green Bay Packers of the 1960s, the San Francisco 49ers of the 1980s and early 1990s and the New England Patriots of the 2000s. What they all have in common great leadership at all levels of the organization. Each organization had a blueprint for success that is laid out in a clear vision by their leader.

MAJOR LEADERSHIP CONCEPTS IN PROFESSIONAL FOOTBALL
Leadership Versus Management

A common misconception is the homogenous comparison of leadership and management. Although these terms have the potential to overlap, they should not necessarily be viewed as synonymous. To put this difference in context, leadership pioneer Warren Bennis was once quoted to say, "Leaders are people who do the right thing; managers are the people who do things right." Teams that succeed do the right thing, all of the time.

Often, a leader is inclined to be invested in interpersonal interaction with others while balancing the organizational vision. With people as a primary purpose, leaders execute decision-making through motivation and inspiration. As a result, the outcome has the tendency to induce change that enables the organization to grow in a positive manner.

A manager is an individual whose work and influence on others is rooted in an assigned role or title. Managers often view productivity and task completion as their primary concerns. As a result of their primary concerns, they carry out ideas through controlling and problem-solving. They do so by formulating strategies, limiting choices, and making the ultimate decisions. With this mindset, results of managerial influences tend to be consistent and predictable.

Although these terms vary, it is important that organizations find a way to integrate both leadership and management to have optimal efficiency and best results. To make exceptional leaders into exceptional managers, it is imperative to find a healthy balance between the positives of each. This aspect of balance is embodied in Blake and Mouton's managerial grid.[4] In this grid, Blake and Mouton provide a simplistic

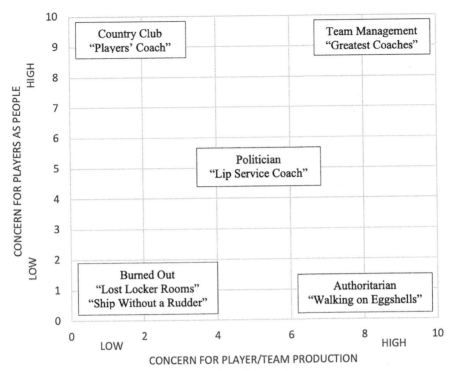

Fig. 1. Managerial grid adapted to football coaching styles.

model of leadership behavior based on production (horizontal axis) and concern for people (vertical axis) based on a 10-point scale. The five styles of leadership outlined include (Fig. 1):

1. 9,1 Authoritarian ("Walking on Egg Shells Around the Locker Room")
   - 9,1 leaders are extremely task-oriented and difficult to work for. There is a notable lack of collaboration, overpowering, and have the tendency to micromanage tasks. Authoritarian leadership causes individuals in the team setting to constantly feel as if they are walking on eggshells and work under a constant veil of fear. In these settings, it is hard to produce at a high level due to the stress and anxiousness of this toxic environment.
2. 1, 9 Country Club ("Player's Coach")
   - This style focuses primarily on people and relationship building while paying little attention to production and output. Some of the characteristics of this type of leader would include being agreeable, actively seeking approval, avoids conflict, and struggles to hold others accountable. Although working or playing for a players' coach may feel good most times, it will not allow for those working for them to optimize their potential to be the best versions of themselves.
3. 5,5 Politician ("Lip Service Coaches")
   - 5,5 leaders operate as the "middle of the pack." They tend to manage situations with a status quo mindset and conform to the opinions of those around them. Politician leaders will tell you what you want to hear to make ends meet. Sometimes coaches that are willing to "toe the line" and lead teams to victories. However, this style is not sustainable and will be exposed over time.

4. 1,1 Burned Out/Impoverished ("Lost Locker rooms" or "A Ship Without a Rudder")
  - This style of leadership lacks commitment to both relationships and performance output. Impoverished leaders take the hands-off approach, remaining neutral in critical situations and meet the bare minimum requirements. Simply, they check the box and collect the paycheck. With a disinterested, apathetic leader, the team culture will organically perish due to the lack of structure and potentiation of power struggles.
5. 9,9 Team Management ("Greatest Coaches")
  - This type of person leads by positive example and fosters a team environment that allows its team members opportunities to reach their highest potential. The focus of this style is to not only develop individuals as team members, but also as people. In this model, leaders are passionate, positive, decisive, and willing to hold the team accountable in a healthy manner. In the sports world, these coaches are the legends that separate themselves from the rest of the pack. They are the type of leaders that regardless of the setting, they would be able to have a positive impact on their organization.

Examples of football coaching styles visualized on Blake and Mouton's managerial grid. Different combinations of a coach's concern for player and team production, as well as their concern for their payers as people create various types of coaches, each with their own benefits and negatives.

Progression of leadership
To be an effective leader, it is imperative that one establishes a healthy balance between the organizational vision and the people they lead. To discover this balance, one must self-reflect throughout their professional journey and identify different techniques that reflect their personalities and help sharpen the focus on what is important. One theory that discusses this growth in a natural progression is John Maxwell's 5 Levels of Leadership model. The five steps are position, permission, production, people development, and the pinnacle of personhood.[5] This is commonly seen in the development of NFL coaching talent. The first step in the development is being placed in a position in which people follow because the formalized role. Once the position is established, the next step is focusing on interpersonal connections and developing relationships. As the relationships strengthen, people gain respect and trust in your abilities as well as the production you bring to the table. As the organization progresses, the next step is developing others into leaders. Once the leader has shown their dedication and investment in the organization, the leader reaches personhood. Personhood can be described as the point in which people follow the leader because of their established reputation.

In football, this progression can be seen when a new head coach accepts the position to lead their new team. Once they are announced, their focus must shift to earning the trust of the locker room and staff members by creating a culture with clearly defined expectations and transparency. As the relationships continue to blossom, the team will be in a position to shift their focus to winning games. When a culture that is rooted in trust is in place, the team will converge as one unit to pursue the common goal of winning a championship. With the buy in of the team and validation of wins, a winning culture is established with a standard of excellence that is clearly defined. With a consistent body of work that includes on field success and a people-oriented culture, legacies are born (**Fig. 2**).

John Maxwell's levels of leadership can be applied to the various levels a football coach progresses through. First, a coach has to fill the open coaching slot and they must earn the trust of their players, which leads to the players buying in and success

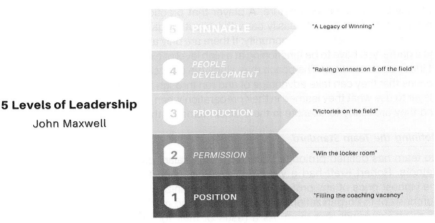

Fig. 2. Five levels of leadership adapted to football coaching styles.

on the field. All coaches are asked to lead their players. The greatest coaches are able to get the most out of their players on and off the field by creating a culture of success.

Lessons Learned from the Greats

Throughout the annals of professional football, there have been an array of coaching, leadership, and mentorship styles that have proven to be successful and consistently result in winning championships. Although there are several ways to achieve a final goal, there are several common threads that all successful organizations have had in common. Some of the major common themes include effective communication, defining the team standard, establishing processes that reflect a vision, and the growth and development of people.

Effective Communication

In the New York Times best-seller book Extreme Ownership: How US Navy SEALs Lead and Win, Jocko Willink notes that "explaining the why and communicating orders in a clear and simple manner greatly enhances the team's performance."[6] Both Vince Lombardi and Bill Walsh were high school teachers and coaches before they became the successful household names we know today. Each of them held the belief that the primary task of a coach was to be an educator. With their educator mindset, they believed in communicating the message to players in a clear, concise manner to ensure the message was effectively delivered.

The book "The Lombardi Rules" outlines 26 principles that Lombardi used to lead the Green Bay Packers to 5 world championships in 9 years. The three ways Lombardi focused on fundamentals were the following:

Build skills: Skills are the building blocks of any organization. You can't put big demands on people before you define and provide the needed skills.[7] Everything begins with the fundamentals and doing the small things right. If you are unable to do these well, then when faced with a crisis situation, such as the final 2 minutes of a close game, then you will not be able to fall back on your fundamentals and your play will be negatively affected.

Rely on repetition: Execution depends on confidence, and confidence depends on preparation. Only after the fundamentals become second nature can you be confident of the results.[7] This results from repetition after repetition until doing the fundamentals properly becomes second nature. A player that practices their fundamentals day in and day out will be able to easily carry these out on game day.

Be prepared to seize the opportunity: If there are only a small number of big plays during a game, you have to be functioning at a high level of excellence to take full advantage of those opportunities.[7] The coach may study the opposing team's film and identify situations that they can take advantage of and run through in practice. This prepares each player to use what they learned in their preparation when the opportunity presents itself, and they are ready to execute in the crucial moments throughout the game.

Defining the Team Standard

No team has defined prolonged success in the salary cap era like the New England Patriots. Robert Kraft had a vision for success when they purchased the team for the highest price of any professional football organization in 1994. Before the Krafts' purchase of the organization, they hovered around mediocrity and were not thought of as an upper-echelon team. As a result of their forward-thinking and leadership, the organization began to flourish. At the completion of the 1999 season, they were faced with a major decision to hire a new coach. They had the vision and foresight to select the best candidate to put them on the path to sustained success. Upon deliberation and outside-the-box thinking, they elected to trade for Bill Belichick. Robert Kraft stated "The greatest decisions I've made in my life are by instinct. I remember when I hired Bill, I had a lot of people telling me it was a mistake. But he and I had established a rapport in "96 when he coached the secondary. You need a coach that understands economics, that understands the impact of the salary cap, and how to make those difficult decisions that allow you to sustain success over the long term. I don't think there's anyone better than Bill at doing that." Like Lombardi and Walsh, Coach Belichick installed a system that was aligned with his beliefs and created "The Patriot Way." Four major tenets of "The Patriot Way" are:

Do your job: Every person in the building has a role and they are expected to do it at their very best. From the players, coaches, and management to the security guards, cleaning staff and everyone in between, each individual understands the importance of their role in fostering and maintaining a championship-caliber organization. Each person should feel appreciated and valued for the job that they do.

Work hard: Preparation is key in professional football. The organization is expected to outwork the competition. The pace is set at the top levels of the organization (ownership and coach) who each lead by example. Within the Patriot Way, the best players on the team are the first ones in the building and are the last ones to leave, always striving to improve with the mindset that no one will work harder than you. When your best players work the hardest, you have great locker room leaders.

Be attentive: Fundamentals are key to any task, if you don't have the fundamentals correct, the mission is destined to breakdown at the most critical situation. Having the fundamentals come as second nature leads to proper execution without thinking, especially in the last few minutes of a tight game.

Put the team first: Every decision is made with the goal of improving the team. A football game is 60 to 70 choreographed plays that rely on 11 players working in unison. If one person does not perform their task properly the team suffers. Players are expected to put the needs and goals of the team ahead of their own individual goals. A highly effective team will thrive if the individual players are willing to put the success of the team ahead of their own personal success.

As stated in the opening paragraph, football is the ultimate team sport which puts a premium on leadership at multiple levels. Leadership is needed from management, coaching staff and most importantly players. To be successful you need your best players to perform at their highest levels in the biggest games. The peer-leadership paradigm of players leading the locker room is the pinnacle of a successful team. This is where peers respond to peers but is one of the most challenging leadership principles to attain. However, once peer leadership is highly functional, there is no stopping the team.

Establishing Processes that Reflect a Vision

When it comes to envisioning and implementing processes inside an organization, Bill Walsh experienced success unlike anyone else. The opening page in his book states, "Running a football franchise is not unlike running any other business: You start first with a structural format and basic philosophy and then find the people that can implement it." Bill Walsh installed his Standards of Performance as a way of doing things, a leadership philosophy, that has as much to do with the core values, principles, and ideals as with blocking, tackling, and passing; and more to do with the mental status than with the physical. Walsh believed if you had the proper processes in place and given the proper leadership that "The Score Takes Care of itself." Joe Montana summarized Walsh's primary leadership assets as follows: his ability to teach people how to think and play in a different much higher, and at times, perfect level. He accomplished these ideals in three distinct ways:[8,9]

1. He had a tremendous knowledge of all aspects of the game and a visionary approach to offense:
2. He brought in a great coaching staff... that adhered to his standards of performance:
3. He taught us to hate mistakes.

Growth and development of people

Bill Walsh truly understood the importance of mentorship through many lessons learned in his life and career. Early in his coaching career, he was an assistant to one of the greatest innovators of his time, Paul Brown. During his time with Brown, Walsh was praised in league circles for his innovative offensive schemes; however, he was not initially hired as a head coach. Even though Brown was his mentor, he was placing his own career development ahead of the loyal Walsh. Brown refused to give Walsh a strong recommendation that would land him a new coaching gig to keep Walsh under his wing and to continue having Walsh as an assistant coach. Walsh vowed to never repeat the treatment he received. As a result, Walsh was instrumental in the career development of multiple assistant coaches that became very successful head coaches in professional football. This is probably one of the best examples of a coaching tree, based upon a successfully led organization. Some of his coaching descendants have made massive impacts on the current game of football, such as Mike Holmgren, who stemmed into Steve Mariucci and Andy Reid; Mike McCarthy, Sean Payton, and John Harbaugh stemmed from Ray Rhodes; and Jeff Fisher who was mentored by George Seifert. The full coaching tree of Bill Walsh that is included below features 10 Super Bowl-winning coaches, a feat no other coaching tree has seen (**Fig. 3**).

Walsh's mentorship philosophy was rooted in a focus on developing independent thinkers. He expected his assistants to aggressively absorb teachings, understand the big picture and adapt to their own philosophic approach.

Medical Team Leadership

Leadership is accomplishing a mission through people. Medical leadership is also an important aspect of the overall ecosystem of a professional football team. The medical team must work in concert with coaches, general managers, administration, staff, and

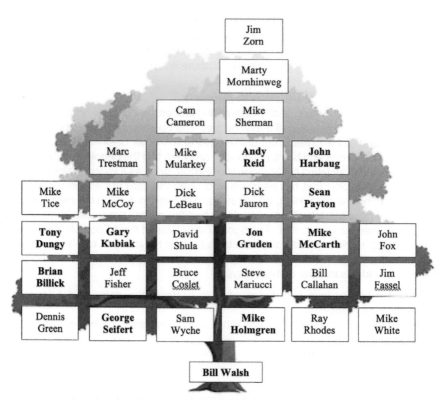

Fig. 3. Bill Walsh's Coaching Tree. This tree represents successful NFL head coaches who coached under Bill Walsh, and successful coaches that they mentored. Together, they have a combined 11 Super Bowl victories and 10 different Super Bowl-winning coaches: George Seifert (2), Gary Kubiak (1), Brian Billick (1), Tony Dungy (1), Mike Holmgren (1), Jon Gruden (1), Andy Reid (1), Mike McCarthy (1), Sean Payton (1), and John Harbaugh (1). These coaches are denoted by bold text.

ownership as leaders of the medical care for the players, as well as the team. This is an important relationship, and to succeed at the highest level, needs to be cultivated with a culture of mutual respect and collaboration. The basic tenet that has to always be at the front and center of the medical team's mindset is player health and safety. This division of the medical team provides the highest level of optimal player health care has to be deeply rooted in the culture of the medical team, so that it can be easily communicated to coaches and team leadership at all times. Medical leadership of a professional sports team is very similar to coaching leadership of a professional sports team. The medical teams vary in size, composition, and structure, as well as organizational behavior and charting, and is very team specific; however basic leadership principles must be adhered to to provide the players with the best medical care possible.

Thus, the medical staff should look to coaching greats, as well as organizations that have exhibited excellence in performance and leadership characteristics to fine tune their medical leadership style. The principles such as leadership accountability, mentorship model, education, and training are applicable, not only to the coaching field, but in medicine and the medical care of the team. Training, repetition, organizational excellence, and expert collaboration, allows for a highly functional medical team, that coexists harmoniously alongside the coaching staff.

In summary, those that have the opportunity to care for a professional, collegiate, high school, or other sports team are entrusted with a special opportunity to not only be embedded with a team, but affect decision-making. The most important aspect for the medical staff is to ensure the health and safety of the athlete. The medical team can learn from the great coaches of our time that have espoused leadership principles of Lombardi, Walsh, and Belichick, and that have consistently taught us the importance of preparation and mastering the fundamentals to do your job well. The team and organizational dynamics are complex and are centered around people first. For a team to achieve its highest potential, leadership at all levels, from peer leadership, all the way to coaching, manager, and ownership leadership is paramount to achieve the vision of a successful organization.

DISCLOSURE

The authors have nothing to disclose about this work. Other disclosures: Dr M.T. Provencher receives royalties from Arthrex, Inc. and Elsevier, Inc., consulting fees from Arthrex, Inc., Joint Restoration Foundation, and SLACK, Inc., and is an honorarium for Arthrosurface. He is currently a Board or Committee member of the following: AAOS: Board or Committee member; AANA: Board or Committee member; AOSSM: Board or Committee member; ASES: Board or Committee member; Arthroscopy: Editorial or governing board; ISAKOS: Board or Committee member; Knee: Editorial or governing board; Orthopedics: Editorial or governing board; San Diego Shoulder Institute: Board or Committee member; SLACK Inc: Editorial or governing board; Society of Military Orthopaedic Surgeons: Board or Committee member.

REFERENCES

1. Pratt M.K., Leadership. In: TechTarget, SearchCIO, Available at: https://www.techtarget.com/searchcio/definition/leadership, 2017. Accessed November 2, 2022.
2. Tzu S. The art of war. Chichester, England: Capstone Publishing; 2010.
3. Kilgore A., Branching Out: Mapping the roots, influences and origins of every active head coach. In: Washington Post, Available at: https://www.washingtonpost.com/graphics/2018/sports/nfl-coaching-trees-connecting-every-active-coach/, 2018. Accessed November 2, 2022.
4. Blake RR, Mouton JS, Bidwell AC. Managerial grid. Adv Management - Off Executive 1962;1(9):12–5.
5. Maxwell JC. The 5 levels of leadership. New York, NY: Center Street; 1960.
6. Willink J, Babin L. Extreme ownership. New York, NY: St Martin's Press; 2015.
7. Lombardi V Jr. The Lombardi Rules. New York, NY: McGraw Hill; 2003. p. 49–50.
8. Walsh B. 1931-2007. The score takes care of itself: my philosophy of leadership. New York: Portfolio; 2010.
9. Beaton A. and Camden H., "The NFL Coaching Tree", Available at: WSJ.com, 2015. Accessed November 2, 2022.

Leadership Lessons Learned from the Military

Francis G. O'Connor, MD, MPH[a],*, Francis H. Kearney[b]

KEYWORDS

- Military leadership • Military decision-making process • Dual agency

KEY POINTS

- Collaboration is the key to interdisciplinary planning and execution.
- Planning, Executing, and Learning as an interdependent team is a critical medical leadership competency.
- As medical leaders, developing medical teams and players is important; having a disciplined structure or process to do so is essential.

INTRODUCTION

Leadership education and training for medical providers has recently been recognized as a core skill in health care that is largely underrepresented in medical education curricula across the country.[1] Health care in the twenty-first century currently demands physician leaders as the medical system confronts several challenges including shifting from a procedure-oriented model to one focused on the prevention and evidence-based management of chronic disease; embracing the challenge of "big data" to improve patient-centered care; increasingly recognizing the role of teamwork in performance improvement; mitigating regulatory burdens that may be obstacles to efficient, high-quality care; and working to address health care inequities.[1-3] The sports medicine community has also identified the need to educate and develop ethical physician leaders with clear challenges to include: ensuring patient confidentiality; promoting an evidence-based return to play guidance; embracing shared clinical decision-making; recognizing the dilemma of dual agency; and finally, promoting the efficacious and ethical management of pain. Recent high-profile sports medicine cases published in the lay press have challenged the public's trust in medical providers, and have reaffirmed the importance to train physician leaders of character.[4,5]

[a] Department of Military and Emergency Medicine, Uniformed Services University of the Helath Sciences, 4301 Jones Bridge Road, Bethesda, MD 201814, USA; [b] Thayer Leadership, 674 Thayer Road, West Point, NY 10996, USA
* Corresponding author.
E-mail address: Francis.oconnor@usuhs.edu

Clin Sports Med 42 (2023) 301–315
https://doi.org/10.1016/j.csm.2022.11.003
0278-5919/23/© 2022 Elsevier Inc. All rights reserved.
sportsmed.theclinics.com

In response to these requirements and gaps, physician leadership education notably has accelerated over the last decade to address these challenges, and assist in developing a new generation of medical leaders.[6,7]

The military provides a valuable resource for the civilian medical education sector to assess, with the intent to potentially model or adopt strategies used to train emerging leaders. The Department of Defense has a long tradition of cultivating leaders, and institutionally invests in the longitudinal education of warfighters. In addition to supporting leadership education, the military espouses a culture that emphasizes and embraces a value system that promotes selfless service and integrity. Although the military services clearly value performance and outcomes, character, leadership, and teamwork are not to be compromised to achieve a result. In addition to leadership training, and a fostered value system, the military additionally trains leaders as staff officers that function as members of a mission-focused team, and uses a defined military decision-making process (MDMP) to achieve the Commander's intent. Finally, the military physician, comparable to the team physician, serves a unique role on a military staff as a both medical provider and as a medical advisor; this role not infrequently presents unique ethical challenges that can be framed in the context of "dual agency.[8]" This article describes the role and challenges of the military medical officer (MMO), and importantly identifies and shares lessons learned in how the military structures and focuses to accomplish the mission, and develops and invests in military leadership training.

A Member of the Military Team: the Physician as an Officer

"There are no secrets to success. It is the result of preparation, hard work, and learning from failure." Colin Powell, former US General, Secretary of State, and National Security Advisor.

General Colin Powell's words in the above quote importantly identify the reality that military success is the result of training and experience. Physicians in the uniformed services are identified on the team as MMOs, and begin the long road of training when they are first commissioned. At Uniformed Services University of the Health Sciences (USUHS), the Nation's only military medical school, academics have attempted to fully define and elucidate the complexity of the unique role of the MMO.[9] The "vector" model of the MMO was first proposed at the USUHS in the early 1990s by then commandant of students, Colonel Barry Wolcott. Dr Wolcott, an emergency medicine physician by training, understood the challenges of developing young MMOs and the value for those officers in providing visualization to help direct and focus their growth.[10] The vector model simply places three primary domains of required skills for the ideal MMO onto the axes of a 3-dimensional graph (**Fig. 1**).

This vector model illustrates the need for the individual to develop a balance of military skills, medical skills, and leadership to become a successful MMO.[10] Effectively developing skills in these three domains ultimately merge them into collective competencies in operational medicine, physicianship, and officership, which defines the professional MMO. These terms, as applied in the vector model, are defined as follows: officership is a set of skills that allows one to function effectively as a leader in the military. Underlying officership are principles, practices, and values that guide judgment, decisions, behavior, philosophy, and vision. Inherent in officership is effective and service-oriented leadership. Physicianship is defined as set of skills that allows the provider to function effectively as a physician with skill in the art of healing. A physician is accordingly educated, clinically experienced, and licensed to practice medicine. Operational medicine adds to standard clinical medicine all

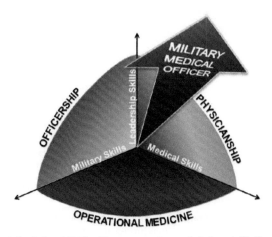

Fig. 1. Vector model of the MMO. (Figure courtesy of Colonel (Retired) Barry Wolcott, Commandant of Students, Uniformed Services University of the Health Sciences, 1892-1993.)

of the unique requirements and challenges of the practicing MMO in the operational and tactical environments, many of which may be nonmedical in nature. This includes a combination of both military and medical skills within the context of the military mission. Although leadership has many components, simply defined, leadership is influencing people by providing purpose, direction, and motivation. Military leadership is further defined as the sum of the qualities of intellect, human understanding, and moral character to enhance the motivations, cognitions, and behaviors of individuals and groups for successful accomplishment of the mission. Finally, operational skills, physicianship, and leadership merge to define and create the professional MMO. Professionalism represents the core of a medical officer's values and behavior and includes personal courage, respect, openness, fairness, empathy, self-improvement, social responsibility, integrity, honor, officership, nonjudgment, altruism, and leadership.

The MMO ultimately functions as a member of a team dedicated to a specific and designated mission. As a member of a team, the MMO functions as a both a leader and as a follower.[11] In the military, in particular in the operational and tactical environments, the physician most commonly functions as a staff officer. Staff operations are well described in miliary doctrine and are service dependent; Army staff operations are detailed in Army Field Manual 6.0 Commander and Staff Organization and Operations.[12] This document details the Army's philosophy of command, emphasizing that mission command is essentially a human endeavor, with successful commanders understanding that leadership guides the development of teams and helps establish mutual trust and shared understanding. The MMO is a vital member of the Command Staff, as is every member of the team. **Table 1** identifies qualities that identify the successful member of a Command Staff (see **Table 1**). These qualities are applicable to both miliary and civilian physicians who function as members of a team. In developing the MMO, these qualities are a focus for continuing education, and additionally assessed through an annual evaluation process.

Military Culture: The Role of the Value System

"Upon the fields of friendly strife are sown the seeds that, upon other fields, on other days will bear the fruits of victory." General Douglas MacArthur.

Table 1
Successful staff member qualities

Successful Staff Member Capabilities	
Characteristic	**Description**
Competent	Effective staff officers are competent in all aspects of their area of expertise. They are experts in doctrine and the processes and procedures associated with the operations process, and they understand the duties of other staff members enough to accomplish coordination both vertically and horizontally.
Initiative	Staff officers exercise individual initiative. They anticipate requirements rather than waiting for instructions. They anticipate what the commander needs to accomplish the mission and prepare answers to potential questions before they are asked.
Critical and creative thinker	Staffs apply critical and creative thinking throughout the operations process to assist commanders in understanding and decision-making. As critical thinkers, staff officers discern truth in situations where direct observation is insufficient, impossible, or impractical. They determine whether adequate justification exists to accept conclusions as true based on a given inference or argument. As creative thinkers, staff officers look at different options to solve problems. They use adaptive approaches (drawing from previous similar circumstances) or innovative approaches (coming up with completely new ideas). In both instances, staff officers use creative thinking to apply imagination and depart from the old way of doing things.
Adaptable	Effective staff officers are adaptive. They recognize and adjust to changing conditions in the operational environment with appropriate, flexible, and timely actions. They rapidly adjust and continuously assess plans, tactics, techniques, and procedures.
Flexible	Staff officers are flexible. They avoid becoming overwhelmed or frustrated by changing requirements and priorities. Commanders may change their minds or redirect the command after receiving additional information or a new mission and may not inform the staff of the reason for a change. Staff officers remain flexible and adjust to any changes. They set priorities when there are more tasks to accomplish than time allows. They learn to manage multiple commitments simultaneously.
Self-confident	Staff officers possess discipline and self-confidence. They understand that all staff work serves the commander, even if the commander rejects the resulting recommendation. Staff officers do not give a "half effort" even if they think the commander will disagree with their recommendations. Alternative and possibly unpopular ideas or points of view assist commanders in making the best possible decisions.
Cooperative	Staff officers are team players. They cooperate with other staff members within and outside the headquarters. This practice contributes to effective collaboration and coordination.
Reflective	Staff officers are reflective in their actions. While conducting actions, they are able to quickly assess and implement corrective measures that lead to successful outcomes. Upon

(*continued on next page*)

Table 1 *(continued)*		
Successful Staff Member Capabilities		
Characteristic	**Description**	
	completion of actions, they analyze and assess events to implement measures that maximize efficiencies in the future.	
Communication	Staff officers communicate clearly and present information orally, in writing, and visually (with charts, graphs, and figures). Staff officers routinely brief individuals and groups. They know and understand briefing techniques that convey complex information in easily understood formats. They can write clear and concise orders, plans, staff studies, staff summaries, and reports.	

Adapted from FM 6.0 Commander and Staff Organization and Operations.

The above quote speaks to the value that then BG Douglas MacArthur saw in those leaders who participated in team sports and later became battlefield leaders in the Army during World War One. It is engraved on the wall in the Arvin Physical Development Center at West Point, NY. The quote reminds us that when General MacArthur was the Superintendent at West Point from 1919 to 1922, he instilled the philosophy that every cadet would be an athlete and participate in sports because team sports developed attributes in those athletes that made them better leaders in combat. The commonalities between sports teams and military teams remain relevant today in our cultures and in the responsibilities military leaders and sports team coaches, physicians and administrators have in holistically developing our soldiers and athletes. Developing future leaders is a core mission for all military leaders to include our military physicians and as such a culture that promotes that notion is critical to success in the military. This core concept is reinforced in a quote from Tayne and colleagues; "regardless of the level of the athlete, interdisciplinary teams will work most effectively when there is a culture focused on shared goals that all work to optimize the highest quality care for the athlete".[13]

Edgar Schein developed the "Iceberg" model for organizational culture.[14] As illustrated in the model, behaviors, rites, and environment are visible artifacts of culture, whereas below the water line, espoused values and underlying assumptions, mindsets, and philosophies as less visible aspects of organizational culture.

A critical component of our Army culture is our values: loyalty, duty, respect, selfless service, honor, integrity, and personal courage, depicted in **Table 2**. An attribute of a values-based culture and critical to successful leadership is trust; in the authors' view, trust is the foundation and cornerstone of leadership. In his book *The Speed of Trust*, Stephen M.R. Covey states that competence and character are the two components of relationship trust; so, leaders and physicians bring their competencies and character to their relationship with their teams and individual players and soldiers, to execute the mission effectively.[15]

Sadly, we have all been witness, in recently publicized cases, to the erosion of trust by athletes who have been abused by team physicians, coaches, and administrators. Similarly in 1996, Army drill sergeants sexually assaulted women recruits in basic training at Aberdeen Proving Ground, Maryland. These examples highlight that espoused values and values in action are sometimes not aligned, which tells us that it is not only critical to have a good culture but we must also work diligently to sustain

Table 2 The army values	
Loyalty	Bear true faith and allegiance to the US Constitution, the Army, your Unit, and other soldiers.
Duty	Fulfill your obligations.
Respect	Treat people as they should be treated.
Selfless-service	Put the welfare of the nation, the army, and your own subordinates before your own.
Honor	Live up to all the army values.
Integrity	Do what's right, legally and morally.
Personal courage	Face fear, danger, or adversity (physical and moral).

that culture. Our current Army values were promulgated after the Aberdeen assaults to invigorate and make ubiquitous values training in our Army. All cultures need sustainment.

Although the benefits of a values-based culture are self-evident, the authors share a story to emphasize the case. The Army's Warrior Ethos is four bullets taken from the Soldier's Creed: I will always place the mission first; I will never accept defeat; I will never quit; and I will never leave a fallen comrade. Creeds are a common artifact in organizations to state the desired values or beliefs. As the nation entered the wars in Afghanistan and Iraq, the Army wanted to focus soldiers with a simple ethos to guide them in the difficult moments of intense combat, which like team competitions hinge on the focused efforts of the team at critical moments.

The story at the video link below is the story of the first living Medal of Honor (MOH) recipient since the Vietnam War, Sergeant Sal Giunta. Sal was a soldier in the senior author (FK) son's company in the 173d Airborne Brigade during their 15-month combat rotation in the Korengal Valley in Afghanistan. Their story is told in a documentary "Restrepo" done by Sebastian Junger and Tim Heatherington and the book War, by the same authors. It is a story of personal courage, loyalty to teammates, duty, selflessness, honor and integrity. It reflects the deep trust the soldiers had in each other and the personal humility of Sal Giunta. The link is a 60 minutes interview between Lara Logan and Sal Giunta and some of his teammates describing the actions for which Sal was awarded the MOH. Rather than a wordy description, watch the video and feel the emotions, trust, and expectations that a trust-based team engenders (**Box 1**).

Our military and sports team cultures are based on trust and on the competence of our teammates and the character they bring to the competition or fight. Without trust you cannot be a great team; so, although purpose, vision and a plan are key elements of success, trust from a great culture provides the winning edge.

Planning: The Military Decision-Making Process

"In preparing for battle I have always found that plans are useless, but planning is indispensable." Dwight D. Eisenhower, 34th President of the United States, and former General of the Army.

"Disciplined Processes Create Agile Organizations." LTG (ret) Frank Kearney, USA

The first quote identified from GEN Eisenhower clearly identifies and recognizes that although the plan may be fallible, the process of planning is critical. The second quote that follows builds on GEN Eisenhower's keen observation. The axiom

<table>
<tr><td>

Box 1
Interview with SGT Sal Giunta

https://www.youtube.com/watch?v=QoEZKyIAPIQ.

13:53 min video, 60 min November 14, 2010 with Lara Logan and SGT Sal Giunta on youtube. com.

</td></tr>
</table>

is a phrase that the senior author (FK) coined as a corollary to a belief espoused by then Joint Special Operations Command commander, MG Pete Schoomaker: "in Special Operations Units we teach people how to think not what to think." We provide frameworks in the military using key processes but the context of 'what to think' is reflective of the individual's operating environment. The US Army philosophy of Mission Command has 7 principles: Competence, Mutual Trust, Shared Understanding, Commander's Intent, Mission Orders, and Disciplined Initiative. This philosophy reflects the complex nature of the battlefields of today and the future, which prevents centralized control during mission execution. Mutual trust is required for this concept to work, as trust underpins the ability of subordinate leaders to exercise disciplined initiative. The Army Operational Model in **Fig. 2** below is simple and effective; leaders plan, leaders prepare, leaders execute and leaders assess and learn.

The Army's planning and decision-making process is the MDMP. Units without a staff use Troop Leading Process; both are shown in **Fig. 3**. After the MDMP is complete, Army organizations rehearse, execute and conduct After Action Reviews (AAR) to assess and learn. These last three steps connect the MDMP to the operations model in **Fig. 4**. MDMP is to plan; rehearsals are to prepare and AARs assess to learn.

MDMP is an adaptation of the five-step problem-solving process taught in high school and college; the military adapted this common process and uses service verbiage and analytical tools as shown below in **Box 2**.

Military culture is a planning culture and planning is continuous and never ending. As identified in the first quote, General of the Army and later President Dwight D. Eisenhower stated" *Plans are worthless, but planning is everything*". This statement means that planning and preparation is key, but plans change routinely based on changes in the environment, on the battlefield or on the court. As the conditions change our plans must be adapted, we fight the enemy not the plan. A plan is static while planning is constant, reactive, and adaptive. So, whether developing battle plans or team strategies or even individual treatment and athlete developmental plans, we cannot be static; we must move at the pace of change.

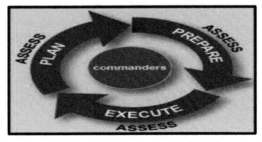

Fig. 2. Army operational model. (*From* Army Doctrinal Publication 5-0, The Operations Process, July 2019, Introduction Figure 1, p vi.)

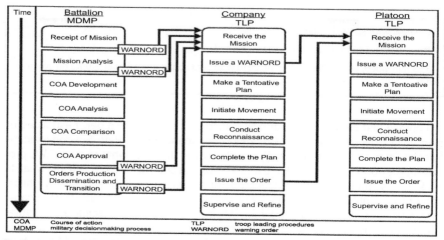

Fig. 3. Army's MDMP and troop-leading process (TLP). (*From* Army Field Manual 5-0, Planning and Orders Production, Department of the Army, 16 May 2022.)

The MDMP is designed for organizations with a robust staff, in the Army that is battalion level and above. Organizations without a formal planning staffs use Troop Leading Procedures (TLP) depicted in **Fig. 3**. TLP are similar to the MDMP but small units don't develop and compare detailed courses of action (COA). Smaller military units get a mission, then assess the situation and develop a hasty plan. These similar processes, MDMP and TLP, are initiated when a new task is directed; the leader initiates planning with his or her Leader's Intent.

Leader's Intent provides the purpose for the mission, the key tasks to be accomplished, and describes what success looks like for the mission. Leader's Intent does not tell the team how to execute the mission but focuses on what the mission is and why we are doing it. Intent empowers innovative solutions, develops

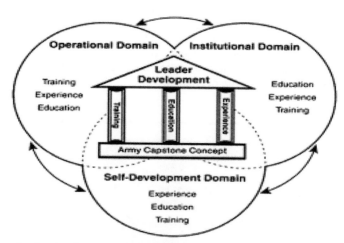

Fig. 4. Army leader development model. (*From* Army Leader Development Strategy 2013, page 8, signed by Raymond Chandler (SMA), Raymond T. Odierno (CSA) and John M. McHugh (SECARMY).)

Box 2	
Problem-solving process and military decision-making process	
Problem Solving Process	**MDMP**
Identify or Define the Problem	Receive the Mission
Gather Facts and Assumptions	Mission Analysis
Develop Possible Solutions	Develop Courses of Action (COA)
Analyze Each Solution	COA Analysis Wargame
Compare Solutions	COA Comparison
Select the Best Solution	COA Approval

subordinate leaders, and recognizes that change on the battlefield is constant. Leader's Intent isn't blind task delegation; a series of brief-backs is required to ensure a common shared understanding of the mission. The first brief-back is a confirmation brief; it occurs shortly after the mission and intent are issued and the team leader assigned the task reflects back what he/she heard and understands the mission and intent to be. The phrase: *I don't know what I said, till you tell me what you heard* is descriptive of why we do confirmation briefs, to achieve clarity of communication and common shared understanding. The second brief-back follows the execution of TLP or MDMP where the executing team briefs the higher commander on how they will accomplish the mission.

During MDMP, Course of Action Analysis and Comparison includes a red teaming process where role players war-game and fight the plan through an action-reaction-counter action process representing the enemy forces, friendly forces, and the operating environment impacts on the plan. Red teaming identifies weaknesses and vulnerabilities and identifies adversary options against which contingency plans can be developed. Once the Course of Action is decided, the plan is published, then the plan and key contingencies are rehearsed. Rehearsals insure a common shared understanding and synchronized execution of the plan as well as lateral accountability among interdependent teams. All players or teams participate in the back-briefs, war games, and rehearsals.

The final process is the most important for military organizations; executing After Action Reviews (AAR) to assess and learn from execution is critical to future success in a continually changing environment. The AAR is a professional discussion involving all members of the planning and executing organizations. It asks and answers four questions: What was the plan? What did we actually execute? What did we learn? and Who else needs to know? If you can answer these questions, focusing on what happened versus who made errors, in a transparent culture, you can really learn about why you succeeded or failed. AARs are not only done in efforts where improvement is needed; they are done when we succeed as well to ensure success is repeatable. The Army and the Joint Military Services maintain extensive databases of lessons learned in the Center of Army Lessons Learned (CALL) and the Joint Universal Lessons Learned (JULL) data center; all new efforts should begin with reviewing lessons learned from past operations.

These processes are common across the military services and standardized for agility. After a few years in the military, these processes are simply *how you think*, just as your clinical procedures and processes guide how your think in medical practice. Ingraining these disciplined processed into an interdisciplinary medical support team, led by the team physician can create the common shared understanding required to guide your planning and execution to enhance successful outcomes and reduce potential errors.

All Physicians Lead: the Military Investment in Leadership Training

You manage things; you lead people. We went overboard on management and forgot about leadership...

—*Rear Admiral Grace Murray Hooper*

Another attribute of United States Army culture is the concept that a core competence for all leaders is to develop the next generation of Army leaders. Every officer in the Army to include our physicians, nurses, physician's assistants, nutritionists, physical therapists, psychologists, and dentists are leaders. Every soldier who remains in the Army after his or her first enlistment is a leader. Therefore, the Army and all military services are in the leader development business, and looking back on my career (FK), I see the leaders I helped to develop as my greatest contribution. The Army Leader Development Model is depicted in **Fig. 4** below.

Three pillars, education, experience, and training operating in three domains: Operational (assignments), Institutional (schools), and Self-Development.

The model in **Fig. 4** applies to officers and noncommissioned officers alike. It focuses on both leadership and management skills in the Institutional and Operational domains; the Self-Development domain is the leader's opportunity to develop complementary competencies or to build on those where he or she needs additional work. Each domain provides the opportunity to be assessed, challenged, and supported to enhance competencies and attributes we expect in our leaders per **Fig. 5** below.

The coaching and mentoring responsibilities for each leader are the responsibilities of their direct leadership. Our efficiency reports are supplemented by routine developmental counseling to support individual development plans for each subordinate leader or soldier. Officers and Army Physicians spend a great deal of time in Institutional Development settings: Non-Medical Corps officers all spend 4 months in a basic officer leadership course (BOLC) to learn their core branch-related skills, 6 months in the Captain's Career course in their 4 to 5 year in service, 10 months as a Major in Intermediate Level Education at the Command and General Staff

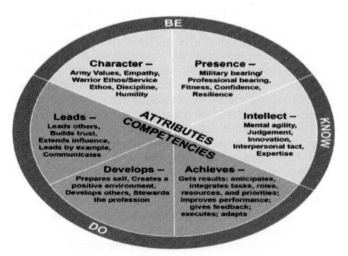

Fig. 5. Army leader attributes and competencies. The army leadership requirements model, army doctrinal publication 6 to 22, army leadership and the profession, November 25, 2019, figure 1–3, page 1-15.

College at Fort Leavenworth or other Service and civilian universities, and 10 months in the War Colleges as Lieutenant Colonels and Colonels earning a Master's Degree in Strategy. General Officers have similar mutli-week courses to develop their senior leader skills.

Our Medical Corp Officers during or following medical school attend a 2- to 14-week service orientation depending on their Military Service requirements. They continue their medical education and licensing and certifications throughout their careers. Physicians also follow the Army Leadership model with assignments in Operational Medicine at Battalion, Brigade, and Division Surgeon levels as well as special Army units and Joint Headquarters. These assignments are either done through permanent duty for a period in the units or through Professional Filler System (PROFIS) assignments where the physician is aligned with a unit that is deployable. The PROFIS doctor would deploy with the unit to major training events and combat assignments. Some medical doctors attend our ILE service schools and our War Colleges. They experience the same operational curriculum as their combat arms and combat support arms peers. They learn and practice the MDMP and AAR processes described in the previous section. The Army expects the same leadership competencies and attributes in them as in all officers; though their focus is their medical competency, they are and must be effective leaders as well.

As an Army doctor, you lead your medical team but each engagement with a soldier is also a leadership mission; you must influence them through purpose, motivation, and direction to follow health protocols, follow treatment and rehabilitation plans and lead healthy lives. To do this, you and your team must have their trust; trust results from demonstrated competency, character and caring. A familiar phrase: *I don't care what you know, till I know that you care* applies. Leading, as a physician, requires time on target with your interdisciplinary medical team and your sports teams; it requires a balance between time in the clinic and time with the troops and athletes. This cannot be achieved by management competencies alone; we must focus on our patients and teams whether soldiers or athletes. Leadership is inherently a people focused endeavor; it requires the same level of deliberate effort required to develop excellence in your medical skills. So, if you let them know that you care, you will garner the trust that allows them to follow your leadership.

Dual Agency: Unique to Military and Team Physicians

"If not you, then who? If not now, then when?" Hillel, 1st Century Jewish Scholar.

The above quote from the Jewish Rabbi Hillel speaks directly to one of the fundamental principles of leadership which is to do the right thing, at the right time. Specifically, the quote is intended to inspire leaders to step up, take action and not wait for someone else to answer the call. This becomes critically important to both military and sports medicine physicians who uniquely confront the dilemma of dual agency, where challenging ethical issues may require difficult decisions. Dual agency, also identified as mixed agency, refers to the conflicts and potential for unethical breaches where a clinician has roles to different entities that may come into conflict for example, an athlete's treating physician with responsibility to the individual, who is also employed by the team, with second responsibility to the team and management.[16] Dilemmas military and civilian sports medicine physicians encounter involve situations in which they face conflicting loyalties (**Box 3**).

The concept of dual agency and ethical issues that confront physicians has been the subject of robust debate.[8] The current military conflicts in the Middle East, in particular, have raised critical concerns with complex issues such as return to duty of individuals on psychotropic medications, forced feeding of prisoners, and "clearing"

Box 3
Dual agency clinical ethical dilemmas

Scenario 1: You are a team physician with a collegiate basketball team trying to qualify for a tournament selection. One of the leading players sustains a head injury with an opposing player with sustaining a brief loss of consciousness. You assess him in the training room and SCAT 5 and VOMS testing is unremarkable. You elect to sit him for the remainder of the game. The coach informs you that he is needed to play in the second half if the team is to have any opportunity to win. The athlete wants to play.

Scenario 2: You are the brigade medical officer on a deployment. A warfighter sustains a brief loss of consciousness during a vehicle roll over incident. Your initial MACE testing is unremarkable, and you elect to place him sick in quarters for 24 hrs. The Commander informs you he is needed this evening on a critical mission for the unit; he is the only member of the team with the required skill set. The warfighter wants to go with the unit.

Abbreviations: MACE, military acute concussion evaluation; SCAT, sport concussion assessment tool; VOMS, vestibular ocular motor screening.

---

individuals for interrogation.[17,18] Although the physician's core ethical construct is to always put the patient first, are there potentially times or scenarios where the mission or team becomes the priority over the Individual? These issues foremost require recognition on the part of the clinician, and an ethical construct for decision-making. At Uniformed Services University (USU), medical students receive hours of dedicated instruction in ethical education. Despite this education, ethical dilemmas will exist and accordingly, the USU is home to the Department of Defense Medical Ethics Center (DMEC) to assist providers.

As illustrated in **Box 2**, decision-making where ethical conflicts may arise, and the medical provider may be asked to place the interests of the team or unit ahead of those of the individual, require an ethical construct. These decisions necessitate that the physician have the requisite training and education in ethical decision-making, and be able to reach out to resources to assist when dilemmas, with no easy answers, require more assistance and guidance. First and foremost, clinician leaders must recognize their potential for dual agency, and the inherent dilemmas in these roles. Recognition in turn should foster discussion, where leaders are often confronted with difficult decisions. Importantly, as identified by Hillel, however, the leader does need to move forward with a decision.

Final Thought: The Stockdale Paradox

"You must never confuse faith that you will prevail in the end—which you can never afford to lose—with the discipline to confront the most brutal facts of your current reality, whatever they might be." Admiral James Stockdale

The nation currently finds itself in an era of challenging times. The slow emergence from the coronavirus disease-2019 (COVID-19) pandemic, current world conflicts, economic downturns, struggles with racial and gender equity, and the often-intense political discourse, can promote a sense of anxiety and hopelessness. Surveys on the world's emotional state have shown a significant impact of COVID-19 on negative emotions, but the increasing level of mental stress is multifactorial. Mental stress and pessimism for the future can be disabling for many individuals, and accordingly, functioning teams. Siegelman has shown that humans are inherently focused on future thinking; he also has devoted a career to positive psychology and the role of optimism.

GEN Colin Powell, in his autobiography, *It Worked for Me, In Life and Leadership*, identifies optimism as a force multiplier.[19] In his final and 13th rules of leadership, he states "Perpetual optimism is a force multiplier." How, however, can we maintain optimism during these challenging times? Another great military leader, Admiral James Stockdale, helps us here, with the "Stockdale Paradox."[20]

The "Stockdale Paradox" was immortalized in the Jim Collins classic text, *Good to Great*.[21] Collins had read Stockdale's memoir of his trials as a prisoner of war in Vietnam for seven-and-a-half years. Collins wondered, "If it feels depressing for me, how on earth did he survive when he was actually there and did not know the end of the story?"

When he posed that question to the admiral, Stockdale answered: "I never lost faith in the end of the story. I never doubted not only that I would get out, but also that I would prevail in the end and turn the experience into the defining event of my life, which, in retrospect, I would not trade." Collins further asked him about the personal characteristics of prisoners who did not make it out of the camps. "The optimists," he replied. "Oh, they were the ones who said, 'We're going to be out by Christmas.' And Christmas would come, and Christmas would go. Then they'd say, 'We're going to be out by Easter.' And Easter would come, and Easter would go. And then Thanksgiving, and then it would be Christmas again. And they died of a broken heart ... This is a very important lesson. You must never confuse faith that you will prevail in the end—which you can never afford to lose—with the discipline to confront the most brutal facts of your current reality, whatever they might be."[20,21]

SUMMARY

The need for physician leaders of character in both the military and civilian settings could never be greater. In this article, we have outlined key lessons that may be learned from how the military values not only leadership as a skill, but perhaps more importantly, heavily invests in leadership education and training; key clinical care points are identified below:

CLINICS CARE POINTS LEARNED FROM MILITARY MEDICINE

- Clinical Point 1: Planning, Executing and Learning as an interdependent team is a critical medical leadership competency.
- Clinical Point 2: As medical leaders, developing medical teams and players is important; having a disciplined structure or process to do so is essential.
- Clinical Point 3: Collaboration is key to interdisciplinary planning and execution; medical leaders need to recognize both leadership and followership roles.
- Clinical Point 4: Trust is the cornerstone of leadership; it is the currency by which we are measured and therefore cannot be compromised.
- Clinical Point 5: Optimism is a Force multiplier; leaders recognize and confront the reality of daily challenges while always projecting confidence and optimism to team members that they will prevail in the end.

We further developed the critical concepts of Mission Command, supported by the disciplined processes of MDMP, TLP and AAR, guided by the 7 principles (Competence, Mutual Trust, Shared Understanding, Leader's Intent, Mission Orders and Disciplined Initiative) operating in a culture of competence, character and caring, to ensure mission accomplishment in ever changing circumstances on the battlefield or on the fields of friendly strife. We additionally explored the challenging role of dual agency as physicians in both military and sports medicine settings need be mindful of ethical challenges that they may confront. Finally, we remember Admiral

Stockdale, and the "Stockdale Paradox;" it is critically important, in particular in these challenging times, that the leader always has faith, and exudes confidence, in the final outcome.

DISCLAIMER

"The opinions and assertions expressed herein are those of the author(s) and do not reflect the official policy or position of the Uniformed Services University of the Health Sciences or the Department; of Defense."

DISCLOSURE

F.G. O'Connor, has no financial interests or relationships to disclose. F.H. Kearney has no financial interests or relationships to disclose.

REFERENCES

1. Rotenstein LS, Huckman RS, Cassel CK. Making Doctors Effective Managers and Leaders: A Matter of Health and Well-Being. Acad Med 2021;96(5):652–4.
2. Rotenstein L, Perez K, Wohler D, et al. Preparing health professions students to lead change. Leadersh Health Serv (Bradf Engl May 7 2019;32(2):182–94.
3. Arroliga ACHC, Myers JD, Dieckert JP, et al. Leadership in health care for the 21st century: challenges and opportunities. Am J Med 2014;127(3):246–9.
4. Belson K. Concussions Doctor Under Scrutiny in Plagiarism Scandal. NY Times. Available at: https://www.nytimes.com/2022/03/21/sports/football/paul-mccrory-plagiarism-concussions.html.
5. Tim Evans MA, Marisa Kwiatkowski. A 20-year toll: 368 gymnasts allege sexual exploitation. IndyStar 2016.
6. Nosé B, Sankey E, Moris D, et al. Leadership training in medicine-12 years of experience from the feagin leadership program. Mil Med 2021;6323377. https://doi.org/10.1093/milmed/usab293 [pii].
7. Frich JC, Brewster AL, Cherlin EJ, et al. Leadership development programs for physicians: a systematic review. J Gen Intern Med 2015;30(5):656–74.
8. Howe EG. Ethical issues regarding mixed agency of military physicians. Soc Sci Med 1986;23(8):803–15.
9. O'Connor FGGN, Kellermann AL, Schoomaker E. Mil Med 2015;180(4):147–52.
10. Woodson J. Roles and Responsbilities of the Military Medical Officer. In: O'Connor FGSE, Smith DC, editors. Fundamentals of military medicine. Borden Institute; 2019.
11. O'Connor FGGN, Harp JB, Deuster PA. Exertion-related illness: the critical roles of leadership and followership. Curr Sports Med Rep 2020;19(1):35–9.
12. FM. 6.0 commander and staff oranization and operations, Military Technical Reource Field Manual.
13. Tayne S, Hutchinson MR, O'Connor FG, et al. Leadership for the Team Physician. Curr Sports Med Rep 2020;19(3):119–23.
14. Schein EH. Organizational culture and leadership. Jossey-Bass Publishers; 1985.
15. Covey SMR. The speed of trust. London, England: Simon & Schuster; 2008.
16. Ray L. The physician's role in modern warfare: an ethical accounting. Virtual Mentor 2007;9(10):663–6.
17. Annas GJ, Crosby S. US military medical ethics in the War on Terror. J R Army Med Corps 2019;165(4):303–6.

18. Annas GJ. Military medical ethics–physician first, last, always. N Engl J Med 2008;359(11):1087–90.
19. Powell CL, Koltz Tony. It worked for me: in life and leadership. 1st edition. Harper-Luxe; 2012.
20. Abrahams BGaR. What the Stockdale paradox tells us about crisis leadership. 2020. Available at: https://blog.sodipress.com/wp-content/uploads/2020/09/What-the-Stockdale-Paradox-Tells-Us-About-Crisis-Leader-HBS.pdf.
21. Collins JGtGRHBB. Good to great. New York: Harper Collins; 2001.

The Highly Reliable, Patient-Centered Sports Medicine Practice

Bruce L. Gillingham, MD, Christopher A. Kurtz, MD*

KEYWORDS

- High-reliability • Resilience • Safety • Patient-centered • Culture • Leadership

KEY POINTS

- In addition to respecting the primacy of the patient's values, beliefs, and desired outcomes in treatment decisions, patient-centered care has as its top priority the delivery of safe, high-quality care. The care team endeavoring to be truly patient-centered will benefit from understanding and applying high-reliability practices to achieve this goal.
- A high-reliability organization (HRO) functions in a complex and hazardous environment like medicine with a much lower rate of mishap and error than expected. The hallmark of an HRO is not that it is error-free, but that it is not disabled by errors. Five key characteristics of HROs have been identified.
- High-reliability behaviors and actions are well shown by high-performing communities in the US Navy. These techniques and practices translate well to the medical environment.
- Optimal performance occurs in a culture that is vigilant and accountable yet strongly supportive of its members. Central to an HRO is a culture that prioritizes safety as its highest ideal. Safety in an HRO is not just a program or a slogan but a central component of the organization's DNA.
- Effective leadership is essential to creating a high-performance, patient-centered care team. In addition to creating a psychologically safe but accountable culture, the leader sets the tone for the team. What the leader values the followers will value. In an HRO, it is critically important that the leader not only set behavioral expectations for the team but also model them.

Since graduating from surgical training 15 years ago, the sports medicine fellowship-trained orthopedic surgeon stands confidently at the operating table. He has hundreds of successful procedures under his belt but is tight on time and anxious to finish this knee arthroscopy quickly so he can grab lunch before his afternoon clinic. Turning to the surgical technician, Jerry Reynolds, a relatively new employee here at the

U.S. Navy Bureau of Medicine & Surgery, 7700 Arlington Boulevard, Falls Church, VA 22042, USA
* Corresponding author.
E-mail address: christopher.a.kurtz.mil@health.mil

Clin Sports Med 42 (2023) 317–324
https://doi.org/10.1016/j.csm.2022.11.004
sportsmed.theclinics.com

ambulatory surgery center, he asks for a scalpel to make his first portal. Reynolds reaches for the 15 blade, but hesitates. Mustering his courage, he says, "But Doctor Banks, we haven't completed the surgical time out." Taken aback, Dr Banks responds, "I don't have time for that. Let's go." Pulse-pounding, Reynolds sees his brief career in the operating room disappearing before his eyes, but he stands firm. "Sir, I am invoking the "two challenge" rule and respectfully requesting that we perform the required time out." Other than the cadence of the anesthesia ventilator, the room falls silent. Stepping away from the table, the surgeon turns and makes eye contact with the technician. "Jerry, you are absolutely correct. Nurse Bowman, as the circulating nurse, would you please read the signed operative permit to verify that we are performing the correct procedure on the correct limb?" Reynolds sags, relieved that he was not ordered to scrub out but even prouder that his voice was heard and that he may have prevented a wrong-site surgery.

INTRODUCTION

In addition to respecting the primacy of the patient's values, beliefs, and desired outcomes in treatment decisions, patient-centered care has as its top priority the delivery of safe, high-quality care. The care team endeavoring to be truly patient-centered will benefit from understanding and applying high-reliability practices to achieve this goal. These are lessons long understood in the US Navy. Navy personnel operate in complex and dangerous environments and yet achieve a remarkable record of safe mission accomplishment. The practices and behaviors they show translate well to the medical environment and offer valuable insights and tools we can profitably apply to the elimination of preventable patient harm and the delivery of patient-centered care. This article outlines the principles and practices of high reliability, illustrate them with examples from operational communities in the US Navy, and show how they can be used to establish a safe, high-quality patient-centered sports medicine practice.

THE FUNDAMENTALS OF HIGH RELIABILITY

As defined by Karl Weick and Kathleen Sutcliffe in their landmark book *Managing the Unexpected*, a high-reliability organization (HRO) is an organization that functions in a complex and hazardous environment like medicine with a much lower rate of mishap and error than expected.[1] The hallmark of an HRO is not that it is error-free, but that it is not disabled by errors. Based on their analysis of several highly reliable organizations –including naval aviation and the nuclear power industry—the authors identified five characteristics defining these organizations, divided into principles of "anticipation" and "containment."

Any team embarking on the journey to high reliability need not look further than the US Navy to find superb examples to emulate.[2] Different parts of the Navy emphasize different facets of high reliability based on the requirements of their unique missions and the lessons they have learned and applied to improve their performance. As in medicine, many of these lessons were learned as the result of tragic mishaps and are "written in blood." Committed to safe, resilient mission accomplishment, the Navy thoroughly reviews these events and adjusts its practices and procedures on an ongoing basis (**Table 1**).

PREOCCUPATION WITH FAILURE

It is important to understand that high reliability is a journey and not a destination and that the patient-centered care team must never be content that it has "all the answers"

Table 1
The five principles of high reliability

Principles of Anticipation	Principles of Containment
Preoccupation with failure and its causes	Commitment to resilience
Reluctance to simplify interpretations	Deference to expertise
Sensitivity to operations	

Adopted from Managing the Unexpected.[1]

nor is it impervious to poor outcomes. Humility is a fundamental characteristic of HROs, which acknowledge and respect the infinite number of ways complex systems can fail. Although it seems counterintuitive, HROs are preoccupied with failure. HROs strive to identify the sources of failure at the lowest possible amplitude to prevent a catastrophic outcome. The ability to anticipate, identify and rapidly resolve variations from normal operations is a defining attribute of an HRO.

High-reliability teams recognize that no matter how carefully they anticipate potential pitfalls, they will still occur particularly in complex systems. Each member of the team remains actively engaged in the work being done and is continually on the lookout for unexpected changes. This requires an active resistance to complacency especially in carrying out routinely successful procedures.

Naval aviation has shown a remarkable safety record despite the hazards of launching and recovering high-speed tactical aircraft in the space-constrained, dynamic, and unforgiving environment of the carrier flight deck. In Naval Aviation, pre-flight briefs are conducted with all members of the flight crew, including the maintenance personnel, to communicate and discuss the flight plan in detail. The team reviews maintenance issues anticipate possible challenges to mission completion and run through procedures to be carried out in an emergency. Clinicians can emulate this practice by holding preop "huddles" with the operating room team to review the surgical plan and required equipment, discussing possible surgical, anesthetic, and nursing challenges, and identifying mitigating strategies to resolve challenges should they occur. This process can be made truly patient-centric by holding the preop huddle in their presence before the administration of anesthetic medication. This practice is also fruitfully applied in the clinic and ward setting to make sure the physician and supporting staff has a shared understanding of the plan for the patients that will be seen, particularly those that present unique challenges or service requirements. This is an opportunity to clarify roles and responsibilities and to optimize care coordination. In the Military Health System, these practices are formalized in the TeamSTEPPS program that has been developed in collaboration with AHRQ (Agency for Healthcare Research and Quality). This evidence-based set of teamwork tools is aimed at optimizing patient outcomes by improving communication and teamwork skills among health care professionals. In the opening vignette, the surgical technician Jerry showed his preoccupation with failure by using a practice termed the "two challenge rule" to overcome the power differential implicit in the operating room. Jerry prevented a potential wrong-site surgery because the culture and system was set up for him to speak up when he observed a deviation from standard practice.

RELUCTANCE TO SIMPLIFY

The next HRO principle is a "reluctance to simplify." HROs are reluctant to simplify or rationalize the interpretation of data that varies from expected normal operations.

Instead, HROs view variances as a window into larger underlying systemic problems. Few organizations are more frequently cited for their track record of safety than the Navy nuclear propulsion program. Underway for more than 60 years without a serious incident involving its nuclear reactors, the Navy nuclear community is a model for producing operational safety in a complex engineering and operational environment. Key to this enviable safety record is scrupulous investigation and resolution of even small changes in reactor operations. A "trust but verify" culture is a central characteristic of the Navy nuclear community and includes close supervisory oversight and two-person verification of data pertaining to reactor operation. Aberrant data is carefully reviewed and a "vertical audit" is performed to assure the integrity of the involved process from top to bottom. "Horizontal audits" that focus on one item across many efforts are performed to validate the integrity of the system as a whole.

Medical teams can profitably adopt these practices by paying close attention to and investigating the cause of any unexpected clinical findings, such as a change in vital signs or unexpected laboratory results. Likewise, the surgical team can "audit" key perioperative steps of the surgical procedure including independent verification of the surgical site and side or the implementation of a "60 s for safety" pause before the completion of the procedure. During the "60 s of safety," all members of the team cease their independent actions and collectively verify the sponge, needle and instrument count, clarify postoperative care requirements, and surface and resolve any team member concerns. Vertical and horizontal audits of any "near misses" that may have occurred during the patient's care should be vigorously pursued as they may identify opportunities to improve the quality and safety of not only the specific procedure involved but the overall care provided by the team. By consistently maintaining a reluctance to simplify and rationalize clinical data and findings that don't meet expected norms the medical team not only improves care for their specific patient but takes the critical first step in identifying and resolving flawed underlying systemic processes that threaten the safety of all patients.

SENSITIVITY TO OPERATIONS

The next principle of high reliability is "sensitivity to operations." Staff members working in an HRO remain actively engaged and sensitive to routine operations, recognizing that complacency is antithetical to safety. This forward-looking mindset is captured in the well-known shipboard mantra that "you can't navigate by your wake." Treating each procedure as a unique event, no matter how routine or frequently performed, is essential to maintaining engagement by all members of the sports medicine team. The use of checklists that require a "challenge-reply" methodology, such as that performed in naval aviation, is a good way to avoid complacency on fundamental but critical steps for safe patient care.

Like naval aviation, naval special warfare (NSW) SEAL teams also have shown unparalleled effectiveness and resilience in consistently completing high-risk missions, such as the Abbottabad raid in Pakistan or the rescue of Captain Richard Phillips from Somali pirates. Although coping with fear and fatigue in deep depths, high altitudes, and dark skies all while facing the very real possibility of hostile enemy fire, NSW operators learn to mitigate risk with checklists, inspections, and extensive training, and mission rehearsals. NSW operators espouse that "amateurs train until they get it right, professionals train until they can't get it wrong."

Arthroscopy simulators and surgical skill laboratories are one-way surgeons can keep their skills sharp and learn to do new procedures before heading to the operating room. For procedures that are particularly complex or novel, rehearsal with the key members of the operating room team either in the skills laboratory or the actual operating room offers not only the opportunity to identify unanticipated procedural challenges and equipment needs but also to increase overall team engagement and effectiveness.

COMMITMENT TO RESILIENCE

Preoccupation with failure, sensitivity to operations, and a reluctance to simplify work synergistically to enable HROs to anticipate and identify potentially harmful deviations from the norm. Committed to resilience HROs are not incapacitated by such deviations. When an error or mishap does occur, HROs are committed to returning the system to normal operations as quickly as possible to prevent or mitigate harm. Practicing the three principles of anticipation described above increases the likelihood that this intervention occurs at a low amplitude before a catastrophic result can occur.

Even so, the most carefully rehearsed operation can still go awry. Navy SEALs prepare for these contingencies as well. For example, despite their meticulous preparation leading up to the Bin Laden raid, one of the two helicopters used to transport the SEAL Team 6 members crashed within his Abbottabad compound. Having anticipated this possibility, additional helicopters were staged nearby and available to replace the damaged helicopter allowing the team to successfully complete the mission.

In the operating room environment, contingency planning is equally important to procedural success. During preoperative planning surgical teams should identify and have a mitigation plan for potential single points of failure. Including alternative implant and instrumentation sets and having them readily available guards against over-reliance on one type of fixation, for example, For procedures that may require other surgical specialists to scrub in, preoperative notification is essential so that this "quick reaction force" is aware and readily available.

DEFERENCE TO EXPERTISE

Another primary mechanism by which HROs achieve resilience is by deferring to subject matter expertise, at whatever level it may reside in the organization. HROs acknowledge that it is impossible to anticipate and prevent all possible failure modes and rely on the active engagement or "mindfulness" of all hands to recognize and intervene when operations do not go as planned. Subject matter experts, doing the actual work "on the deck plates," are often the most aware of small, subtle deviations from normal operations and the interventions necessary to address them. Engagement by all members of the team, each of whom is obligated to speak up if he or she recognizes a deviation from the established procedure, is an essential counterweight to the most common source of error-—human factors. In Naval aviation, for example, it is estimated that 85% of mishaps are due to human factors.[3] Recognizing the potentially intimidating effect of differences in rank and qualification level, aviation procedures empower all members of the crew to speak up when it is their judgment that additional critical information needs to be considered. These procedures are known as "aviation crew resource management" and provide formal rules and procedures that foster engagement and shared responsibility by all members of the team.

This "egalitarian vigilance" also is a hallmark of NSW. Dive buddies check each other's equipment and jump masters inspect everyone's parachutes and regardless of rank, all platoon members are obligated to alert their teammates if they see something wrong. Having all members of the patient care team participate in Team-STEPPS program training or a similar crew resource management curriculum is an effective way to instill active engagement and mindfulness in all personnel and will accelerate the team's high-reliability journey. Rotating the leadership of the preop huddle among all members of the operating room team encourages them to understand the procedure more holistically and fosters active engagement beyond the member's primary role.

THE IMPORTANCE OF CULTURE

Optimal fleet performance occurs in a culture that is vigilant and accountable yet strongly supportive of its members. Central to an HRO is a culture that prioritizes safety as its highest ideal. Safety in an HRO is not just a program or a slogan but a central component of the organization's DNA. Insisting on high ethical and performance standards makes it easier to identify deviation from expected norms. Effective leaders invest the time to identify the strengths of the individual crew members and then place them in positions to maximize their strengths. For example, special warfare leaders know that even though not everyone has the skill and aptitude to become a sniper, they can fulfill other mission-critical roles. In the medical setting time taken to carefully interview new members of the team by asking open-ended questions and truly listening for their strengths and unique abilities is time well spent.

In an HRO, leaders must establish a safe environment for engagement by all members of the team. Even when incorrect, input by all personnel, especially those most junior or newest to the team, should be acknowledged and discussed. This is the basis for the egalitarian vigilance that is critical to high reliability and is one way to create an environment of high-velocity learning. Every engaged sailor is an additional "sensor" monitoring the complex operational environment for unexpected and potentially dangerous variations. An environment of psychological safety also makes it easier for a crew member to ask for help and to have his request viewed as a sign of strength rather than a weakness.

LEADERSHIP ESSENTIALS

Effective leadership is essential to creating a high-performance, patient-centered care team. In addition to creating a psychologically safe but accountable culture, the leader sets the tone for the team. What the leader values the followers will value. In an HRO, it is critically important that the leader not only set behavioral expectations for the team but also model them. She must show a preoccupation with the sources of failure, insist on not normalizing deviance from expected operations, remains situationally attuned to current operation no matter how routine, and actively avoid complacency. When an error or mishap does occur, the leader should openly acknowledge it and show confidence in the ability of all members of the team to contribute to resolving the issue to minimize harm to the patient. HRO leaders make it clear that they are never content and are constantly seeking to improve both their own and the team's performance to optimize patient outcomes.

Naval aviators perform a post-flight "debrief" immediately following mission completion to identify opportunities to improve squadron performance. Members of the team figuratively "leave their rank at the door" to encourage open, honest discussion. The leader is not immune to criticism and more junior team members are required to report deviations from the flight plan by any of the involved pilots. Taking the time to perform a postoperative or end-of-the-day clinic huddle, particularly when events did not go as planned, is an important way to capture lessons learned before important nuances and insights are lost (**Table 2**).

Table 2
High reliabilty principles in action: applying fleet best practices to the medical arena

HRO Principle	Fleet Best Practices	Medical Applications
Preoccupation with failure	Pre-flight briefs	Preop and Preclinic huddles
Reluctance to simplify interpretations	Horizontal and vertical audits Two-person verification	Universal protocol Surgical "time out" 60 s for safety
Sensitivity to operations	Challenge-reply checklists Training and rehearsals	Rehearsal of complex procedures Surgical skills labs
Commitment to resilience	Contingency planning Quick reaction forces	Back-up surgical sets Subspecialists on standby
Deference to expertise	Crew resource management Egalitarian vigilance	TeamSTEPPS® mindfulness

SUMMARY

Practicing safe, high-quality patient-centered care is challenging. Fortunately, valuable insights are gained by observing HROs such as those seen within the US Navy. Be it the disciplined engineering of the nuclear submarine force, the choreography of naval aviation on an aircraft flight deck, or the elite teamwork shown by the SEALs—examples abound that can be profitably translated to the medical environment. Leaders who invest the time and energy to create the appropriate culture and who understand and model the required behaviors for their teams will enjoy an exponential return on their investment in terms of professional satisfaction and the delivery of truly patient-centered, safe, high-quality care.

CLINICS CARE POINTS

- Listen to your team members when they speak up. They may be correct in pointing out a potential deviation from safety. Even if incorrect, ask yourself why they thought that. It is an opportunity for learning and they may not be the only team member who misunderstands.

- When something is not as it should be, pay attention to it. Resist the temptation to write-off unexpected adverse events. Oversimplification as "one-offs" allows those events to multiply and recur.

- When it comes to patient safety and quality, set rank, title, and position at the door. Recognize the expertise of every team member and leverage all of their strengths.

- If you think you may need something if even unlikely, then have it available. Resiliency is built upon preparedness.

Lead by example. High Reliability is a culture. The leader sets the standard

DISCLOSURE

The authors certify that they have NO affiliations with or involvement in any organization or entity with any financial interest or nonfinancial interest in the subject matter or materials discussed in this article. The views expressed are those of the authors and do not reflect the official policy or position of the US Navy, the Department of Defense, or the US Government.

REFERENCES

1. Weick KE, Sutcliff KM. Managing the unexpected. San Francisco (CA): Jossey-Bass; 2001.
2. Gillingham B, Corbridge J, Warner H, et al. Fleet practices are driving better health care. Proceedings 2016;10:42–7.
3. Dunn RF. Discovering human factors. In: Gear up, mishaps down: the evolution of naval aviation safety, 1950-2000. Annapolis: Naval Institute Press; 2017. p. 89.

Coaching in Sports Medicine

F. Winston Gwathmey, MD*, Mark D. Miller, MD

KEYWORDS

- Coaching • Mentorship • Orthopedic education

KEY POINTS

- Coaching is common in sports and many other professions.
- Teaching and mentorship is fundamental in surgical career development. Surgeon coaching is not as common.
- Widespread utilization of surgeon coaching is impeded by several factors including cost, time constraints, lack of perceived need, and surgeon culture.
- Surgeon coaching should be expanded in orthopedic surgery and sports medicine, in particular, to optimize performance.

As the end of my fellowship approached in 2013, I had the opportunity to sit down with Dr Atul Gawande in his office at Brigham and Women's Hospital in Boston with my fellowship mentor, Dr Thomas Gill, to discuss surgeon coaching. Dr Gawande, who had risen to prominence with his best-selling books *Complications* and *The Checklist Manifesto*, had introduced the concept of surgeon coaching in an article in the New Yorker the previous year.[1] My residency mentor, Dr Mark Miller, was the program director for the upcoming 2013 annual meeting of the American Orthopaedic Society for Sports Medicine (AOSSM), and had planned a session on coaching in sports medicine. Dr Miller thought that the Gawande video interview would be a perfect addition to that session given his expertise on the subject.[2]

Dr Gawande recounted an experience he had on a tennis court several years prior in which a superior player had given him helpful tips while he soundly defeated him. He improved several facets of his game just by being coached on his technique by another tennis player. Watching a professional tennis match soon after that experience, he noticed that even the top players in the world have coaches who provide constant, real-time feedback. It occurred to Dr Gawande that surgeons are not so different from elite athletes. Surgeons possess an elite skillset that is constantly put to the test with challenging operative cases similar to how an athlete's skillset is put to the test during competition. However, surgeons do not use a coach to optimize their technique and provide feedback about areas for improvement.

Department of Orthopaedic Surgery, University of Virginia, University of Virginia Health System, 2280 Ivy Road, Admin South, Charlottesville, VA 22903, USA
* Corresponding author.
E-mail address: fwg7d@hscmail.mcc.virginia.edu

Clin Sports Med 42 (2023) 325–333
https://doi.org/10.1016/j.csm.2022.12.005
0278-5919/23/© 2022 Elsevier Inc. All rights reserved.
sportsmed.theclinics.com

Building on his experience on the tennis court, Dr Gawande decided to apply the coaching concept to his performance in the operating room. He invited a retired former attending from his residency program to observe him in action during surgery. A postoperative debriefing was insightful for Dr Gawande as his coach catalogued several areas for improvement ranging from draping adjustments to changing how he held his instruments. These seemingly inconsequential behaviors collectively decreased the efficiency of the operation and the performance of Dr Gawande and his assistants. The behaviors had evolved and crystalized over time in large part due to lack of feedback. Coaching made a positive difference.

Sport medicine surgeon coaching was featured at the annual meeting of the AOSSM later that summer.[2] In addition to the Gawande's recorded interview, 2 surgeon coaching teams presented their experiences as part of the symposium—one from San Antonio, Texas, and one from North Carolina. The San Antonio team consisted of Dr Brad Tolin (surgeon) and Dr Jesse DeLee (coach), and the coaching occurred in both the clinic and the operating room. The coaching objective in clinic was to evaluate patient flow and efficiency in the delivery of service. An outside set of eyes proved to be invaluable as Dr DeLee identified several systems issues and offered suggestions for improvement. In the operating room, the goal was to elevate the efficiency of surgery. Again, Dr DeLee brought a new perspective on many seemingly minor aspects of the operating room set-up that optimized Dr Tolin's team. Drs DeLee and Tolin created an action plan to address these issues and ultimately found the experience to be extremely eye-opening and helpful.

Dr Dean Taylor (surgeon) and Dr Walt Curl (coach) were the participants on the North Carolina team. They brought a similar approach to the exercise with observation in both the clinic and operating room. The feedback session started off with "what is working" and Dr Curl outlined several areas in the clinic that seemed to improve function and efficiency. A preclinic "huddle" with the clinical staff, physicians, and students was identified as a particularly useful exercise. Dr Curl then enumerated his thoughts for improvement and highlighted strategies for dealing with frustrations. In the operating room, Dr Curl focused on preparation for surgery and teaching of residents and students. At the end of the visit, Dr Taylor had acquired numerous tips and tricks for improving performance in both the clinic and the operating room.

Both coaching teams reported an unequivocally positive experience. Coaching illuminated "blind spots" in a surgeon's clinical and operative practice that an outside eye could more readily appreciate. The experience also prompted surgeon introspection into personal performance and the strengths and weaknesses of the system in which he was practicing orthopedic sports medicine. Ultimately, the coaching exercise led to an overall improvement of the practice. The teams emphasized the importance of selecting the right coach for the surgeon. The coach needed to have an understanding of the type of practice, patient population, and operative cases to impart meaningful analysis. Specific problem areas should be preidentified to maximize the efficacy and efficiency of the coaching process. Both teams concluded that coaching in sports medicine should be expanded. However, nearly a decade later, there has been little development in the realm of surgeon coaching in orthopedic sports medicine.

Medical education is a lifelong process of continuous learning. The field of medicine is constantly evolving and physicians must keep pace with the science to provide appropriate care to patients. The surgical education system is built on a foundation established more than a century ago by Sir William Osler and Dr William Halsted at Johns Hopkins University hospital.[3] Surgeon teachers and mentors were central to this system in which trainees would care for surgical patients under the direct supervision of a practicing surgeon. Surgical residency and fellowship programs have flourished under this preceptorship model since its inception. However, the transition from training to independent practice presents a challenging and treacherous time for a developing surgeon because the direct supervision abruptly disappears. The newly independent surgeon must rely on his or her training and funds of knowledge to provide appropriate patient care. Steps that were simple during training suddenly seem more complex and uncertain with no direct feedback from an experienced faculty. Additionally, a newly independent surgeon may be working in a practice and hospital setting with staff that may be unfamiliar with the types of cases he or she plans to perform. Building a practice can be an uncomfortable and inefficient process. The strength of a surgeon's teaching and mentorship can facilitate that process.

Teaching, mentorship, and coaching have overlapping characteristics, and a surgeon can function as a teacher, mentor, and coach simultaneously[4] (**Table 1**). The mode of information sharing in each of these categories is different. Teaching imparts foundational skills and concepts to the novice learner. Mentorship expands on teaching to incorporate practice development, career support, and professional advice.[4] Mentorship often occurs over the course of a longer term relationship between the teacher and learner. Although teaching and mentorship incorporate active transmission of information, surgeon coaching consists of observation of performance, analysis, surgeon reflection, and implementation of feedback. Progression from novice to expert follows a gradual transition from teaching to coaching. Louridas and colleagues[5] proposed that the 2 techniques used by surgeons to improve performance lie on a continuum with teaching involving the directive transfer of information for skill acquisition and coaching involving nondirective self-reflection for skill refinement. The development of expertise is a strenuous process and should not follow the misguided historical mantra of "see one, do one, teach one."

Training surgeons are coached throughout residency and fellowship and receive copious real-time feedback from their attending surgeons. Practicing surgeons are not afforded that same real-time feedback despite the fact that most surgeons continue to develop expertise throughout the duration of their surgical practice. Continuing medical education and surgical skills courses are processes by which practicing surgeons can stay up-to-date and acquire new skills. Practicing surgeon performance is broadly monitored by patient satisfaction, outcomes, and performance measures. However, the critical evaluation of surgical performance and the feedback mechanism central to the training process do not routinely occur.

Surgeon coaching has received increasing attention recently due to the clear potential improvement in surgeon performance and the resulting patient care benefits. Continuing medical education for orthopedic surgeons historically has involved attending specialty-specific conferences. However, a review of the impact of continuing education for health professionals demonstrates only a modest improvement in patient outcomes.[6] Higher intensity interaction in an educational setting has been proposed to have a more significant impact on the improvement of performance for the health professional.[7] Extensive research of elite performers has identified deliberate practice and critical feedback to be essential for the acquisition of expertise.[8] Newly independent surgeon has acquired the basic skillset to perform the surgeries he or she learned during training. However, to attain an expert level of performance, additional skill growth is necessary. The development of an expert skillset comes with repetition, experience, and personal introspection. Surgeon coaching has the potential to expedite this process. Coaching has also been proposed as means to improve surgeon well-being, increase resilience, and reduce burnout among surgeons.[9]

Table 1

Teaching, mentoring, and coaching in surgery

	Medical Student	Resident	Fellow	Junior Faculty
Teaching	History and physical examinations Patient presentations Basic surgical skills	Patient management Specialty-specific surgical skills	Advanced patient management Advanced surgical skills	Complex patient management and multidisciplinary approaches New techniques
Mentoring	Career options Application guidance Networking Research involvement	Career paths Specialty-specific networking Research presentations	Job search Contract advice Society involvement	Building practice Research collaboration Local and national committees
Coaching	Providing constructive feedback Encouragement Technical practice	Clinical scenarios Surgical technique feedback Surgical simulation Mock oral examination	Complex clinical case discussions Surgical technique feedback Surgical simulation Mock oral examination	Clinic flow and opportunities for improvement Operating team/room setup Surgical technique feedback

Surgeon coaching comes in many forms. Lin and Reddy described 2 types of coaches: expert coaches and peer coaches.[4] An expert or instructional coach is an experienced surgeon who helps a learner change practice through self-assessment and constructive feedback. This type of coach is specifically useful to help a surgeon acquire a new skill or procedure. A peer coach has a similar level of experience and the feedback is more bidirectional. This type of coach helps to optimize practice habits and promote surgeon introspection into performance. Most descriptions of surgical coaching involve one surgeon visiting and observing the other and providing in person feedback. In this scenario, the surgeon identifies areas in which feedback and data collection would be helpful. The coach observes, collects requested information, and facilitates the reflective conversation at the end of the visit. Technological advances have created the ability for remote coaching through video streaming. The coronavirus disease 2019 pandemic prompted the proliferation of telemedicine and exposed most surgeons to the capabilities of videoconferencing for patient care. Telementoring has been proposed as a technique by which experienced surgeons can guide learners through complex surgical cases remotely through video streaming.[10,11]

A recent systematic review of 26 articles about surgeon coaching demonstrated overwhelming support for the benefits of coaching with high rates of positive change in clinical practice directly associated with coaching.[12] In a survey of 521 surgeons with a variety of backgrounds and experience levels, 84% responded that they would be willing to participate in a peer coaching program. Most of the respondents indicated that coaching in the operating room would be the most useful approach. A systematic review of coaching to enhance surgeons' operative performance demonstrated that surgical coaching interventions had a positive impact on learners' perception and attitudes, technical and nontechnical skills, and performance measures.[13] A statewide coaching program targeting intraoperative performance of bariatric surgeons in Michigan received favorable reviews from the participants and decreased operative times.[14] Despite the obvious benefits of and interest in surgeon coaching, the actual utilization of surgeon coaching remains very low.

Many obstacles have been described that prevent the routine utilization of surgeon coaching.[4,7,15,16] The clear obstacles to the routine utilization of surgeon coaching is logistical constraints, expense, and the opportunity cost of lost clinical practice time. It is not practical or financially attractive for an experienced surgeon to take time away from his or her practice to visit another surgeon. Additionally, some surgeons do not see the need and report a perceived lack of benefit as a reason not to pursue physician coaching. Surgeon culture has also been described as a barrier to surgical coaching as surgeons value their image of competence and autonomy. Many surgeons feel threatened by the concept of surgeon coaching with significant concerns about the impact on their reputation.[4]

Models of successful surgeon coaching programs have been developed. The Wisconsin Surgical Coaching Framework was created as a formal program that defined core competencies for surgical coaching.[15,17] According to this program, coaching for surgeons can target performance improvement in 3 domains: (1) technical skill, (2) cognitive skill, and (3) nontechnical skill. Three distinct but interrelated activities of coaching were defined as follows: (1) setting goals, (2) encouraging and motivating, and (3) developing and guiding. In setting goals, the coach and participant should recognize the ability and experience of the surgeon, build rapport and trust, and define appropriate and achievable goals of the coaching plan. The coach should encourage and motivate the participant by active listening, support, promotion, affirmation, and inspiration. The coach should challenge the participant during the process. The coach develops and guides by providing directive feedback, asking questions, modeling, informing, confirming, and providing counsel and advice. The coaching program should optimize the controllable components such as selection of an effective coaching and careful design of the coaching context.

Surgeon coaching has established a strong foothold in several surgical realms such as general surgery, urology, and obstetrics and gynecology. However, surgeon coaching in orthopedic surgery has not been as widely pursued, in large part, due to the obstacles inherent the practice. Surgeon coaching in orthopedics, however, has been proposed as a tool to promote a passion for performance improvement as well as a method to decrease burnout. Orthopedic trauma surgeon Dr Jeffrey Smith writes about the value of coaching in orthopedic surgery.[18] He defines his "8 Practices of Highly Successful Surgeons" (**Box 1**). He writes high-performance surgeons engage in coaching to maintain or reinvigorate that passion for performance improvement in anything and everything. Dr Smith confronted his own issues with burnout by pursuing formal coaching training and now runs a national surgeon coaching program.

There is a logical connection between coaching and orthopedic sports medicine because no other surgical specialty has as close a relationship with athletics. The orthopedic sports medicine surgeon often coaches an athlete through injury, recovery, and return to play and communicates frequently with athletic trainers, coaches, and parents. Despite the robust mentorship network within the orthopedic sports medicine field, surgeon coaching in sports medicine continues to be an underutilized tool. Most practicing sports medicine surgeons attend educational conferences and surgical skills courses to maintain competency and learn new techniques. There are also programs in which practicing sports medicine surgeons can visit expert surgeons to observe surgical procedures. Surgeon coaching, in which an expert or more experienced surgeon visits and "coaches" another surgeon, is not a routine practice. Many of the previously outlined obstacles to surgeon coaching are present within the field of sports medicine. Logistical issues, cost, and culture may be deterrents to pursuing surgical coaching. There may also be a stigma that surgeon coaching represents some type of remediation. However, the notable potential benefits cited by the surgeon coaching teams who presented at the AOSSM Annual Meeting would lead to the conclusion that expansion of surgical coaching the field of sports medicine would be a fruitful endeavor.

Perhaps, the biggest obstacle to the adoption of surgeon coaching in orthopedic sports medicine is the lack of awareness of the possibilities of surgeon coaching. Surgeons may also lack insight that they would benefit from an outside set of eyes to optimize their practice and individual performance. The cost of surgeon coaching may seem to outweigh any potential benefit. With the ever-growing emphasis on patient

---

Box 1
Eight practices of highly successful surgeons

- Passion for performance improvement
- Reciprocity of roles and relationships
- Attitude resilience
- Communication with mutual understanding
- Time/life management using rhythm
- Inspiring to shared goals
- Complex problem solving through simplicity
- Energy for personal and practice wellness.

outcomes, patient satisfaction, and productivity, there is reason to think that surgeon coaching to improve performance will gain momentum. There is a growing body of research that demonstrates the inherent value of surgeon coaching due to reduced operative times, increased surgeon efficiency, and improved patient experience. It may be the responsibility of the orthopedic sports medicine societies and hospital systems to normalize and promote the concept of surgeon coaching for widespread adoption to occur.

For surgeon coaching to work in orthopedic sports medicine, an effective and reproducible program must be established. Smith lists 10 elements to successfully establishing a surgeon coaching program (**Box 2**).[18] For an orthopedic sports medicine coaching program to be successful, the participating surgeon must concede to being coachable. It may be difficult for the surgeon who is considered the expert in his domain at the hospital to allow an outsider to critically analyze his practice. Self-reflection and introspection may not be comfortable but the vast majority of surgeons who participate in a coaching find considerable value in the exercise. The surgeon coaching teams of Taylor/Curl and Tolin/DeLee stressed the importance of selecting the right coach for the surgeon. The surgeon should have some familiarity with the type of patients and cases a participating surgeon performs or else the feedback may not be as useful or relevant. Additionally, the specific goals of a coaching session should be reviewed in advance so that the process is efficient and problem focused.

Finding appropriate and effective coaches would seem to be an obstacle to establishing a successful sports medicine coach program. Expert sports medicine surgeons have their own careers and taking time away from practice is costly and onerous. Retired or part-time surgeons represent a potential cache of coaches that could form the foundation of a surgeon coaching program.[19] A recent survey of more than 2000 retired general surgeons showed more than 50% of respondents were interested in surgeon coaching with 82% willing to mentor for free.[20] Orthopedic sports medicine societies could survey retired surgeons in their memberships to create surgeon coaching pools. Interested surgeons could submit coaching requests within these pools and matched with an appropriate coach. Video "telecoaching" is also an area

---

Box 2
Ten elements to successfully establishing a surgeon coaching program

- Create buy-in from stakeholders (ie, administration, participant surgeon)—there needs to be perceived value and/or incentive for the program to be viable.

- The purpose and goals of the program need to be identified—will coaching improve surgical performance, wellness, team building, and so forth?

- Develop the program purpose, mission, vision, and foundational principles and ensure alignment with the organizational structure and culture.

- Establish and measure desired outcomes—objective benefit such as improvement in career satisfaction, patient satisfaction, safety, or risk abatement should be measurable.

- Establish budget, infrastructure, resources, and time.

- Define clear expectations, roles, and responsibilities for the program leaders, coaches, and participating surgeons.

- Train coaches internally or hire coaches externally.

- Educate surgeons in best practices of coaching.

- Commit to provide value to each surgeon and remove barriers to participation.

- Assign appropriate coaches for participating surgeons.

ripe for exploration with the advancement of video streaming and videoconferencing capabilities.[10] Hospitals and surgery centers could develop methods to allow expert surgeons to observe surgical procedures and provide real-time feedback to the surgeon and operating room staff to improve performance.

Most surgeons would agree that they are better at surgery now than they were 5 years ago. This improvement in skillset is developed through learning, experience, and reflection. They figure out what works and what does not work and modify technique based somewhat on trial-and-error. This does not seem to be the most efficient process to refine a skillset. An observer with the expertise to critically analyze that surgeon could facilitate the recognition of areas for improvement and enhance skill acquisition and performance. When an athlete seeks to improve performance and add skills, a coach is central to that process. It would make sense that a surgeon could benefit from a similar approach.

CLINICS CARE POINTS

- Demonstrated benefits of surgeon coaching include improved clinical and surgical efficiency, reduced cost, improved physician wellness, reduced surgeon burnout, and better patient outcomes.
- Successful surgeon coaching implementation requires planning including establishing value and/or incentive in the program, clear expectations, and appropriate coaches for participating surgeons.
- Obstacles to surgeon coaching include logistical issues, cost, and culture.
- Society and institutional support may be required to drive widespread surgeon coaching in sports medicine.

DISCLOSURE

The authors have nothing to disclose related to this article.

REFERENCES

1. Gawande A., Annals of Medicine, Personal Best, Top athletes and singers have coaches. Should you? The New Yorker, 10-3-2011, Available at: http://www.newyorker.com/reporting/2011/10/03/111003fa_fact_gawande.   Accessed August 10, 2022.
2. Gawande A, Taylor DC, Curl W, DeLee JC, Tolin BS. Symposium – Improving your game – surgeons coaching surgeons. American Orthopaedic Society for Sports Medicine Annual Meeting. July 2013.
3. Kerr B, O'Leary JP. The training of the surgeon: Dr. Halsted's greatest legacy. Am Surg 1999;65(11):1101–2.
4. Lin J, Reddy RM. Teaching, mentorship, and coaching in surgical education. Thorac Surg Clin 2019;29(3):311–20.
5. Louridas M, Sachdeva AK, Yuen A, et al. Coaching in surgical education: a systematic review. Ann Surg 2022;275(1):80–4.
6. Umble KE, Cervero RM. Impact studies in continuing education for health professionals. A critique of the research syntheses. Eval Health Prof 1996;19(2):148–74.
7. Zahid A, Hong J, Young CJ. Coaching experts: applications to surgeons and continuing professional development. Surg Innov 2018;25(1):77–80.

8. Ericsson KA, Lehmann AC. Expert and exceptional performance: evidence of maximal adaptation to task constraints. Annu Rev Psychol 1996;47:273–305.

9. Dyrbye LN, Gill PR, Satele DV, et al. Professional coaching and surgeon well-being. A randomized controlled trial. Ann Surg 2022. https://doi.org/10.1097/SLA.0000000000005678.

10. Gerardo R, Lele P, Sundaram K, et al. Surgical telementoring: Feasibility, applicability, and how to. J Surg Oncol 2021;124(2):241–5.

11. Greenberg CC, Dombrowski J, Dimick JB. Video-based surgical coaching: an emerging approach to performance improvement. JAMA Surg 2016;151(3):282–3.

12. Valanci-Aroesty S, Alhassan N, Feldman LS, et al. Implementation and Effectiveness of Coaching for Surgeons in Practice - A Mixed Studies Systematic Review. J Surg Educ 2020;77(4):837–53.

13. Min H, Morales DR, Orgill D, et al. Systematic review of coaching to enhance surgeons' operative performance. Surgery 2015;158(5):1168–91.

14. Greenberg CC, Byrnes ME, Engler TA, et al. Association of a Statewide Surgical Coaching Program With Clinical Outcomes and Surgeon Perceptions. Ann Surg 2021;273(6):1034–9.

15. Greenberg CC, Ghousseini HN, Pavuluri Quamme SR, et al. Surgical coaching for individual performance improvement. Ann Surg 2015;261(1):32–4.

16. Beasley HL, Ghousseini HN, Wiegmann DA, et al. Strategies for Building Peer Surgical Coaching Relationships. JAMA Surg 2017;152(4):e165540.

17. Vande Walle KA, Quamme SRP, Beasley HL, et al. Development and assessment of the wisconsin surgical coaching rubric. JAMA Surg 2020;155(6):486–92.

18. Smith JM. Surgeon coaching: why and how. J Pediatr Orthop 2020;40(Suppl 1):S33–7.

19. Kim NE, Moseley JM, O'Neal P, et al. Retired surgeons as mentors for surgical training graduates entering practice: an underutilized resource. Ann Surg 2021;273(3):613–7.

20. Valanci-Aroesty S, Feldman LS, Fiore JF Jr, et al. Considerations for designing and implementing a surgical peer coaching program: an international survey. Surg Endosc 2022;36(6):4593–601.